Relearning to speak after a stroke:

A step-by-step guide on regaining your speech after a stroke.

A Simple Self - Help Guide to Regaining Speech

Ashvin Mohindra
FCILT, MBA, MSc, MRes, MCIPS

Copyright © *Ashvin Mohindra*, 2025
All Rights Reserved

This book is subject to the condition that no part of this book is to be reproduced, transmitted in any form or means; electronic or mechanical, stored in a retrieval system, photocopied, recorded, scanned, or otherwise. Any of these actions require the proper written permission of the author.

This book is dedicated to my family, Remi, Ella, Raj, Kalpana, and my mum, who have given me hope, guidance, and support throughout my recovery journey. I am profoundly grateful to you all for your love, unwavering faith, and encouragement.

Author Background

My name is Ashvin Mohindra. I'm a 54-year-old, well-educated man who has worked in the supply chain, logistics, and procurement sectors for over 30 years, creating end-to-end service solutions. I regard myself as young at heart.

I had a difficult upbringing, starting from a very young age. I understood early on that life is hard and that you can only expect good outcomes if you work for them. Managing personal and professional targets and relationships was key to my success.

Growing up and living around Heathrow, I was connected with many service delivery firms with connections with supply chain and logistics organisations. I was taught to manage projects and processes and think in an organised and systematic way. I worked up from shop floor operations roles to senior upper management positions. Luckily, I was mentored by powerful men and women who taught me how to understand the micro and macro world and border systems that affect me directly and indirectly.

I met my wife at university when we were in our twenties. I had our first child (Ella) when I was 34 and our second child (Remi - son) when I was 40. They are my world. They are at the top of every personal list and my number one priority. So much so that I have reorganised my life to be present there for all their life events; as teenagers, they have the answers to every question in the world; however, with more parent-experienced eyes, one can see that they both need more structure, time, guidance, love and time to mature.

I've had two major heart operations and two major strokes. I'm newly divorced. I chose to end my 27-year relationship (about 3 years ago) when my health continued to change from bad to worse.

Before having serious health issues, I had traditional views of relationships. I was that husband who worked long hours to create a large house filled with "things" for my family but never allocated time for me and always put my children's and wife's needs in front of mine. I was a provider. I was always aware of business issues but never invested time to learn about myself and lacked self and relationship awareness to help my marriage.

I have two brothers and one sister who have achieved remarkable professional success, working as coroners, doctors, barristers, judges, business consultants, teachers, and so on. In short, I am surrounded by overachievers who are highly competitive, critical, and profound thinkers. These are typical traits of the successful individuals I know. Our personal suffering and struggles have instilled significant character, attitude, and resilience. Being surrounded by people of this calibre is exceptional, and their qualities influence each of us.

The primary drawback of surrounding oneself with an exceptionally intelligent family is that everyone has an opinion. Being in the company of knowledgeable individuals constantly challenges your beliefs, values, and thought processes, facilitating rapid growth and agility. How we think as a family is typical for us; however, it is a double-edged sword. On one hand, superior knowledge does not guarantee that individuals possess the soft skills necessary to navigate relationships effectively. Furthermore, everyone tends to be competitive and desires to 'win,' preferring to discuss subjects where they have expertise. Conversely, it can be observed that family relationships among intelligent individuals can be highly beneficial, as the sharing of knowledge and ideas fosters an excellent environment for growth and enhancing one's understanding of the world. When one of us encounters a challenge, we all come together to share the issue and support one another in resolving our problems. My perspective is that our family's superpower lies in our ability to unite; we each bring different viewpoints on how to support one another, which encourages us to grow beyond the capabilities of other families.

Over my 35-year working life, to help me connect multi-level skills with individuals, I have chosen to work to simplify my relationships, communication, lexicon, and the language around me, from industry buzzwords to more simply understood words and meanings.

Five years ago, in November 2009, just before the start of COVID closures, I had just finished my MBA and was working as a consultant in procurement when I was diagnosed with heart failure. One of my high-pressure heart valves was failing, and the doctors gave me six months to live. My heart was working at around 70% functionally and had dropped normally expected. Rather than worry or burden my wife and children (who were doing their exams or too young to understand) with my health condition, I made the painful decision not to tell them that I have an issue with my heart, as I did not want my health issues to interfere with their activities; school/studies and their lives. I was stuck in the hospital for around a month, and I was subject to many tests and regular monitoring. I agreed with the hospital that if they allowed me out for Christmas, I would take it easy and not exert myself in any way. A follow-up appointment was scheduled for early Jan.

At my first appointment in January 2010, I was told my mitral heart valve was failing faster than expected, and it was down to around 20%. The doctors then told me that the initial 6 months to live had been cut to less than 3 months at best. - I chose to keep this information to myself once again, aware that my daughter's essential exams at the age of sixteen were approaching in May, and I didn't want to add to her concerns. Any reasonable parent or father would make the same decision; they would prefer to endure any pain or suffering rather than pass it on to their children.

Luckily, I was supported by my eldest brother Raj, who was a consultant cardiologist and a barrister, who translated the doctor's speech into easy language so I could make informed decisions about my care and explore my options for dying. I had to face my demise, and I had a lot of hard conversations and coming to terms with my end-of-life decisions. This was a dark time, and I had to project a smiling, supporting face to my children and wife whilst keeping my pain hidden from them. I wanted my children to remember who I was and not pity or feel sorry for me as they watched me die slowly. – I watched my father die this way, and it broke me, and I wanted to save my children from this painful journey.

When anyone gets the news that their life has been shorter, or when a person places a clock on their life, it will floor them: shock or disbelief, denial, anger, bargaining, guilt, depression, and acceptance and hope. I was the same. My glass-half-full attitude changed to a half-empty one. My thoughts were very dark indeed, and I needed a way to distract myself from my looming demise. This was my time to make the hard choices about the life I wanted and on what terms I wanted to accept. I went through the various stages of grief and emotions, and as learned from the movie The Green Mile, with the epic saying, "I guess it comes down to a simple choice: get busy living or busy dying". I chose to get busy living.

Once my tears had dried, I reflected on my problem-solving skills and fight-or-flight options… knowing that I had never given up on a task or test, the choice was evident: I would go down fighting and on my own terms, as I was not about to abandon myself or my children. I needed to alter my attitude and perspective to survive while staying true to my own principles.

At this point, I reflected on my experiences and knowledge. I began to question every boundary imposed on me, both professionally and personally, that could apply to every direct and indirect structure, infrastructure, and process I knew or understood. I hoped that someone might provide me with Answers. I had too much time on my hands and needed to manage my time and activities more effectively.

Surprisingly, over the years of facing challenging tasks, people, and environments, I taught myself to adopt a half-full-glass perspective rather than a glass-half-empty outlook. To simplify, I do not resolve my heart or physical issues, but I can focus on utilising my energies to enhance my mental health. Firstly, I needed a personal desire to change, one that would provide me with purpose and hope. Secondly, I required distractions from the health issues I could not control. I must take ownership of my actions and decisions and refrain from blaming others.

Playing chess is featured regularly within my family, and we all understand that to conquer your opponent, you must first understand them. I need to understand myself, my weaknesses, and my strengths, take accountability for my situation, and not adopt a victim attitude. I needed to own my new life and my disabilities. The battle with my mind and knowledge began. With a renewed desire to recover, I decided to consider the future and started to reprogram my thinking. Mentally, I was convinced that I would live longer than the 3 months given to me by the doctors; I had beaten longer odds before in a professional capacity. I would reapply this mental reprogramming to my personal growing thinking.

With a failing body and little physical strength, I knew I had to keep my mind sharp and focused, and I needed clear goals that I could control. My goal was to reach the top of my industry, as I hoped to return to work soon. To achieve these aims, I enrolled in three master's level challenges: supply chain, procurement, and logistics, hoping that I could defy the odds and live longer than the three months given to me and that I would pass all of the educational challenges. If I survived, my target was my personal prize: I wanted to emerge as a leader in the supply chain industry, so I used my study and upskilling time constructively.

I was in and out of hospital for years, monitored closely and regularly. I attended online classes, but I was alive and scheduled for a heart operation at the Royal Hospital in London.

On the day of my first heart operation and in the days that followed, I was placed in the ICU in an induced coma for a couple of days to give my heart time to recover. The initial heart valve operation was a success.

Within days, I was moved back to the cardio ward to recover. Two days after I emerged from the coma, the on-call registrar visited me. The doctor attempted to remove the pacemaker. They pulled the pacemaker wires so forcefully (instead of cutting them) from my chest that they tore a larger hole in the exterior of my heart. While I was awake, I felt the blood drain from my heart, and I had an out-of-body experience where I saw and sensed the doctors cutting me open as they operated on my heart for the second time, just days after the first major operation. I died for approximately four and a half minutes.

Once more, I found myself back in the ICU, placed in an induced coma for approximately a week. The hospital was uncertain whether I would survive. Upon awakening, I was left with only one functioning lung; struggling to breathe was a new low, even for me. I was receiving dedicated morphine. Yet, I was still alive, having defied the long odds again, and I began to appreciate the value of air. I had never valued breathing or air until this experience.

Living with and recovering from a major heart issue is one thing, but undergoing two back-to-back major heart surgeries within days of each other is extremely rare. Both the inside and outside of my heart had been compromised, and the doctors informed me that I had approximately 12 years to live.

Within two days, my second lung reflated, and I breathed independently without supplemental oxygen. A few days later, the hospital transferred me to another facility, where the doctors put me on a rigorous course of blood thinners that caused nosebleeds lasting 6 to 8 hours each.

Around 2-3 weeks, I was discharged from the hospital and sent home.

I was a picture; my scars looked very scary, and I looked like a shark had attacked me, and I was covered with bandages and plasters that covered every part of my chest. On my side table was a never-ending big bottle of morphine and various other medicines. If I could jump up, I'm sure I would have rattled.

My son Remi was an excellent support during a time when one of my lungs was significantly damaged, and my heart felt incredibly sore. Remi helped me exercise by taking slow walks around the house and in the garden. It took me over a month to venture beyond my home. I still needed to rest to recover and catch my breath every few paces. He was patient and always encouraged me to take my time while cheering me on. Additionally, Raj was my sounding board, guiding me like a compass when I felt lost and needed direction and strength.

A couple of weeks after my daughter's exams finished, I sat both of my children down and explained the truth about what had happened to me and why I had concealed my complex, serious health issues from them. This was a difficult conversation for our family; I felt it was essential to be honest with them. Watching my son's face as he cried upon receiving the news was heartbreaking for me, yet my children understood my reasons.

Up to now, I had no control over the external health events I had to endure. All I knew was that I had a hereditary heart problem inherited from my father, and I had survived. At that time, I was informed that my life expectancy was shortened, and I could expect to live no more than 12 years. I was determined that some good would arise from this grave situation.

Over the past years, I have had plenty of free time and wanted to keep my mind active, so I completed various courses. I was also awarded a Fellowship in Logistics and master's degrees in Procurement, Supply Chain, and Logistics. Additionally, I mentored master's students online until I had my first stroke.

Observing my relationships and those of others and realising that my life operates on a clock dedicated to my actions, I have come to understand that life is "not a dress rehearsal." I have realised that to improve myself, I must invest in cultivating my self-awareness and understanding of relationships, as well as in developing and sharing my knowledge more broadly.

Teaching stroke survivors to communicate from first principles is not addressed anywhere online or in any book. This book will fill that gap in the market, and more importantly, it will assist others in improving their speech and enhancing their comprehension. It is delivered, combining numerous books, articles, and the latest scientific research into a simple, structured framework that offers long-term support for patients and "supporters" (caregivers, doctors, nurses, or hospitals).

When I had my stroke and lost the ability to talk, my children had the time to help me. This book is written to appeal to supporters of all ages and skill levels (caregivers, nurses, doctors, etc).

(If you wish to donate to assist me in setting up an app to help others enhance their speech, search for this title online.)

My only constants are my love for my children and my thirst to improve myself and the world.

Table of Contents

Author Background 1
1. Why and how to use this book? 11
2. Stroke (Brain Injury) Day 17
3. Awakening 20
4. Tiredness 23
   4.1 Vitamins 24
5. Attitude 26
   5.1. Healing from past traumas 30
6. Stages of Grief 33
7. What are the major types of strokes? 35
8. Speech Symptoms 37
   8.1 Aphasia and apraxia 37
      Key points about aphasia 37
   8.2 Dyspraxia 38
9. Current Speech Framework 39
10. Areas of Brain Function 42
11. Easy Framework: "How to speak again." 46
    11.1 Recording Ability Progress 47
12. Stage 1: Physical Issues 48
    12.1 How to recover? 48
    12.2 Abilities to track 49
13. Stage 2: Pictures, Films & Gestures 50
    13.1 Pictures & Films 50
    13.2 Gestures 51
    13.3 Abilities to track 51
14. Stage 3: Letters, Words, & Numbers 52
    14.1 Letters 52
    14.2 Letter & Words 53
    14.3 Numbers 64
    13.2 Abilities to track 65
15. Stage 4: Reading & Spoken 66
    15.1 Abilities to track 69

16.	Useful apps	70
17.	How to Improve Comprehension	72
18.	Tracking Speech & Comprehension	74
17.1	How to use the table	76
19.	Overview of Comprehension	78
20.	Effects of CBD and THC	80
20.1	CBD	80
21.2	THC	80
21.	Organisational Support/tools	82
21.1	Infrastructure Performance Guide	82
21.2	Nurse Performance Measurement	83
21.3	Stroke metrics to monitor the recovery of patients	84
22.	Creating Analysis to Measure Performance & Quality	86
22.1	Diagnostic analysis	86
22.2	Descriptive analysis	88
22.3	Predictive analysis	90
22.4	Prescriptive analysis	92
23.	Brain Care	94
23.1	Calcium	94
23.2	Plaque	94
23.3	Microplastics	95
23.4	Water	96
23.5	Must-have foods	97
24.	Gifts	99
25.	Conclusion	101
26.	List of Tips	106
27.	Tracking Speech & Comprehension - Template	114
28.	References	117

1. Why and how to use this book?

This book is about my journey to teaching myself to talk again after the medical staff had dismissed me and what I learned from my experiences after having a significant stroke or brain injury. It differs from all other books on developing speech and comprehension skills by putting the patient's journey at the heart of the book. The book also shares the input from the support staff (doctors, nurses, and support staff) and the organisations that deliver the speech services.

My experiences will highlight the difference between the current administered treatments by approach organisations in a top-down method vs. a bottom-up approach, which firstly prioritises the patient's outcome. - The top-down approach benefits medical organisations/hospitals first. Its overarching priority is saving money, whereas the bottom-up approach prioritises patient outcomes.

As a person who has experienced two strokes, I found that the current books and papers target medical professionals or patients. When I had my first stroke, my teenage children and adults were unable to assist me as there were no simple books available for purchase that could aid non-medically trained individuals in helping themselves. This book addresses the gap in the market for "teach yourself to speak again" literature following a stroke or brain injury.

This book aims to reach and help as many people as possible with brain injuries that have affected their speech and their support staff, doctors, and organisations that provide support services to their recovery.

The book, by design, aims to appeal to as broad an audience as possible, so I shall utilise fewer medical terms and more straightforward language to convey my ideas and experiences. I will write this book using common, accessible words instead of incorporating all the global research and knowledge gathered in its creation. Yes, this means that research references will be provided at the end of the book. I anticipated that having these references might be rather dull for most readers, so I have chosen to write this book without in-text citations, omitting all the "heavy" medical terminology while including essential medical terms that patients will encounter during their recovery.

This book differs from many other available titles. It delves into the topic of recovering speech after a brain injury, an area that only a few doctors and patients have truly explored. Based on my research, no one has authored a book that combines the perspectives of patients, doctors, support staff, and organisations that assist stroke and brain injury victims in helping them understand the various pathways that aid in regaining speech. The book presents the easy-to-apply pathways and methods for patients to restore their speech. It's important to note that the author suffered a severe stroke, resulting in the loss of speech, and subsequently taught themselves to speak again when the hospitals had given up on me. (I have first-hand experience of losing my speech and, as I often say, "I have skin in this game.")

I have over 30 years of experience designing, creating, buying, selling, and managing blue-chip supply chain services, and my unique skill set is well-suited for writing this self-help book.

I will detail my experiences, from first having a stroke and will highlight the current research and share my speech experiences with other professionals/experts who deliver stroke recovery services.

Every year, there are over 80k people in the UK; in the US, there are approximately. 900k people have a stroke each year. Of these, just under 78% have a speech issue directly attributable to their stroke. (Around 10 million people are affected each decade in the UK and the US only.)

For most people who have a stroke, it affects their speech directly for most people with speech issues that have risen from strokes. Many do not get their speech back in full, and no long-term support is available to help them. Generally, the speech recovery stats from strokes are abysmal. Speech support groups that I have attained focus on talking therapies and not on upskilling the patients and the support staff to help the patients reintegrate into society.

To put these stats into context, they indicate that over the last decade, only approximately 8-9 million people in the USA and UK who previously spoke without an issue now have speech issues that have arisen from strokes. This means that between the US and the UK, around 8 million people will have long-term problems with their speech. This number is magnified sizably when tracked over the same period and across more countries. – This affects the patient's chances of returning to work and drains our economy.

Strokes can be viewed as a primary compounding societal problem. Currently, in the two trusts in Surrey, UK, that I have engaged in for this research, I see that the hospital patient's physical and spoken recovery is tracked at a basic level only, and their services are at the hospital door. Patients' development and delivery of speech services are fragmented, disjoined, not monitored, tracked, and personalised for the patients and the hospitals (who deliver their services to the patients). The idea I suggest is that this will be a record that can be followed by the person in and out of the hospital so macro and micro monitoring can be achieved. Once we understand standard service, we can improve and scale the services and save money simultaneously.

Patients often ask why governments or medical stroke service providers have not tackled this issue as a whole rather than split the treatments into the following issue areas:

1. The physical treatments are varied; many do not involve pathways that help patients recover completely.

2. In outdated frameworks, Current speech treatments are basic and complex to follow or understand.

3. Post-stroke comprehension issues can affect the brain's ability to process speech.

4. Doctors' appetites and frequency for working together or sharing new practices can be slow and hit-and-miss. They focus on their speciality areas of skills and do not venture beyond them.

5. New treatments must be more standardised and centrally administered; therefore, tracking patients' and doctors' progress and trends is often overlooked.

6. Doctors and support staff base their knowledge on the research they read about, not the feedback of stroke survivors. All hospital systems follow a similar approach that is inflexible and does not address all of the issues that affect patients. A combined top-down and bottom-up approach is required to evolve from the current top-down teaching direction to a bidirectional one.

Currently, there are no worldwide agreed post-stroke speech treatments that target speech improvement. No globally agreed post-stroke speech treatment framework has been devised that can be applied to post-stroke survivors to help patients improve their speech. It is beneficial to recognise that addressing all stakeholders' interests, e.g. hospitals, remote support services, etc., and providing consistent speech and/or treatments for brain injury survivors. It is a challenge for most organisations. Specifically, the structures of departments and frameworks that the staff use are outdated and do not provide long-term patient planning.

(** It has to be pointed out that hospitals are business first. Secondly, they are there to deliver services and treatments as cheaply as possible, whenever possible. One must map and measure the progress and performance before understanding it. - If a hospital cannot charge/profit for a service/pill, why would it offer their service? It is a business first.

A reasonable argument can be made that suggests that hospitals/institutions do operate and follow guidelines when it suits them. However, if there are no metrics to measure speech recovery performance, how can the hospitals measure the performance of the patient/s, support staff, and the hospitals/institutions and their efficiency? Currently, no simple, easy-to-understand, end-to-end long-term speech recovery pathways are available. – I have included the current speech recovery framework and have created an updated, much easier framework that simplifies the recovery pathways and can be followed by the patient on their end-to-end journey. (It can be used by people aged 10 and older.)

Hospitals want to charge for as much as they can get away with. Treating speech recoveries is a low-cost and low-return service as the treatments are hard to follow and administer.) - Being aware of why hospitals do not develop long-term therapies and who is gaining but not developing treatments.

From my experience within NHS (Surrey) stroke departments and online dedicated stroke groups, organisations and their staff generally focus on physical treatments, addressing the patient's physical recovery only and overlooking the patient's speech challenges. Short—and long-term speech recovery rates are usually abysmal. If hospital trusts and organisations cannot define what "good looks like" in service delivery, then how can they improve outcomes?

Speech issues are generally classified into two primary groups: issues that one is born with or develops over one's life.

This book will examine all the major available speech processes, expand on them, and include an updated speech-learning framework I created from my experience as a stroke survivor. This framework will give you insights into my recovery journey, the pathways I used, and what works and why it works. I will provide the reader with an overview of the recovery stages and include many tips I learned from my journey. This framework is presented as an easy-to-follow and monitor development program.

I have consolidated almost all the key research and boiled it into a more simplified, structured way to understand the subject without overly jargon-laden medical terms. I will share the currently used framework and propose a more uncomplicated and straightforward framework for helping survivors improve their condition. The current books on regaining speech are written by doctors who have never had strokes, have book knowledge but no direct speech, have lost personal experience, or are patients who lack medical knowledge. The book proposes how to manage a speech department efficiently and cost-effectively. This book is laid out in a point-by-point pathway that can help any reader or patient improve their speech after a brain injury. I have also added a step-by-step process for teaching and tracking others' attempts to speak again. (This will standardise the monitoring and treatment of recovers.)

This book combines the most current knowledge and thinking of various stakeholder groups and their views.

I have included many learning "aids" I used to regain my speech and highlighted what worked for me on my path to speaking again. I had to experience various treatments and medicines, and I will share what worked, what did not, and why.

Currently, there is no long-term practice of monitoring or targeting patient speech improvement. Patients' recoveries are at a significant disadvantage because they are overly focused on physical recovery and lack an easy-to-follow speech recovery framework or mechanism that can be shared.

Using the updated framework and tips, you/support staff/organisations can monitor/track the patient's progress in a structured scientific way. This approach will improve patient outcomes, help monitor patients, shorten recovery times, make processes more efficient, and save money by improving efficiency. Pathways have from having a stroke and would have significantly reduced my speech re-learning time. It will also examine the order of treatments provided to me by the UK medical staff and hospitals and suggest a more structured, standardised way to help patients. - The updated speech framework will discuss what treatments worked, how they affected my recovery, and how you can take charge of your own long-term recovery. This framework will speed up your speech recovery.

If you know people who have had strokes/brain injuries and have speech issues, or if you treat or support the patients/recoveries, then this book is for you.

2. Stroke (Brain Injury) Day

I was a Global Supply Chain Procurement Consultant who lived with my wife and two teenage children in Surrey, England. By nice, I mean it is close to good schools, excellent hospitals, great outdoor areas to have fun and explore, etc. In short, it's a great place to raise children and enjoy family time.

Our extended 5-bedroom house is big enough to be lost in. My friends call it a "sizable place."

To understand my values, it is essential to know that my family consisted of immigrants from Kenya who settled in England in the 1960s. I grew up in a very modest, working-class family that held middle and upper-class values. The core principles we were taught included valuing education, respecting everyone, and believing in karma. My father explained that my role was to embody "good" in all its forms. I recall vividly when he told me that my responsibility was to pass on what I had learned to my children and that we all share a duty to make the world a better place for everyone.

I now have to explain that I am British Indian, and my ex-wife is English, and many of our worldviews differ. In practice, we have agreed on roles and expectations of each other. However, our different values have a source of strength and also our problem.

On Saturday, July 5th, it was early morning, a sunny morning. My teenage children were playing music, playing on their iPhones, and watching TikToks while my wife busied herself upstairs doing her admin in the study.

I tended to the garden tasks: mowing the lawn, clearing the drains, and so forth. That morning, I had not eaten or drunk anything, as I wanted to get an early start on the day since I had a lot of work to complete. The morning was predicted to be quite hot.

I came in from the back garden and made my way to the kitchen to fetch a glass of water. I rushed through the back door, and my headache grew more intense and painful. I began to feel dizzy and light-headed. My thoughts sparkled as though fireworks were erupting in my head. In my mind, I could see white flashes illuminating the veins in my brain, each vein glowing white with a blue halo encircling it. The background colour of my mental vision was a deep, blood red. A few seconds after these symptoms emerged, my legs buckled beneath me, and I found myself sprawled on the downstairs floor, shouting for help from my family.

I dragged myself through the kitchen and lay on the floor alone. My family were upstairs, and I was downstairs. It was about a minute before they heard my cry for help and came downstairs to find me on the floor, struggling to speak or stand. I banged on the kitchen radiator to raise the alarm.

In the semi-conscious state, my body began to curl up into the foetal position as my brain shut off the areas of my brain that were starved of blood or nourishment. The feeling can be only described as someone who is switching areas of my brain. With no control of my brain or body, my body and bowls relaxed… I shit myself.

My son Remi was the first person to come downstairs, and he saw me lying on the floor, asking for help. I drifted into and out of consciousness. My wife called the emergency services, and my daughter comforted me by holding my hand. When my mind was present, I understood her and asked for help, explaining my feelings and situation. – Intermittently, I lost all control of my body and of my mind.

Luckily, an ambulance turned up within 10 minutes, and they diagnosed me as having a stroke. They lifted me onto a stretcher, and under blue lights, they transported me to the nearby hospital emergency department.

To summarise my position with you, I'm back in hospital again. My health has taken a downturn to a new low and is plagued by blood clots stemming from various heart operations. I found myself in a hospital bed, having lost all ability to speak, write, and communicate.

I was partially disabled both physically and mentally, and I was drifting in and out of consciousness. I was scheduled to have an MRI to scan my brain. I was making sense in my mind, but no one could understand any words coming out of my mouth. I could not write or communicate as my right side (face, arm, hand and foot) was not responding. This was my brain shutting down the affected parts of my brain that were being starved of blood. The brain was rerouting signals that would keep me functioning on a fundamental level only. Simply put, my brain put me in pure "survival mode" as my brain tried to reboot itself.

The MRI showed that I had a brain clot (ischemic) and not a brain leak (haemorrhagic) stroke. This is lucky, as my type of stroke could be treated by clot-buster medicine and no drilling was required. – Had I had a brain leak stroke, then the doctors would have located it and then treated it by drilling into my skull to treat the leak.

Every stroke is personal and differs from person to person. The location of the issue within the brain, the size of the clot, diet, gender, race, and other factors can all change the symptoms and outcomes for each person. The speed of initiation of diagnosis and then treatment is key.

My last memory is of being parked outside the MRI department in a cold hallway. I passed out for what felt like hours, watching the fireworks explode in my mind: a stream of shooting blues, red and white tracers, and stars that crackled in my thoughts.

3. Awakening

When I woke up, my surroundings had changed. I had been moved into a stroke ward within the hospital. Nothing was familiar. No one was there to talk to me or explain where I was, what had happened, and what I could and could not do. I was terrified. The first thing I noticed was that I had an extreme headache, and I was very sensitive to all sounds.

I lay on the bed, confused and disoriented, moving between being awake and unconscious. I had never had a headache before, yet now I had the most severe headache that I have ever had, and my thoughts were still playing this firework show in my brain. This was a terrifying time for me as, just like that, my thoughts and perception of the world changed. The world as I know it was unfamiliar to me. I had lost all the film of memories, and my thoughts were limited to pictures only.

I further noticed I could not focus on anything for less than a few seconds. I could not talk or make sounds. It was like someone had turned up the volume of my sensors: my touch, my sounds, my inability to process questions or find answers. Processing my thoughts (sounds, words and sentences) was difficult. To frame this re-awaking environment in a hospital, there are sounds from machines, alarms, bleeps from monitors, people talking, etc., and they surround me everywhere. And every tone or sound hurt my brain. The light hurt my eyes and my brain. I found that keeping my eyes closed and covering my ears was the only way to minimise the pain.

A nurse came to tell me that I had a stroke. However, I could not talk. I could not make any sounds at all. When I tried to spell or write a word, I could no longer spell, write or count. I tried to control my hands but could not do this well either. I struggled to hold a pen and found it challenging to draw a straight line. I could not communicate. I had difficulty pointing at things and making gestures.

I then tried to test my other senses. My right lower arm and hand were affected. My hand was "clawed," and I could not open it. I had lost feeling in the lower parts of my right leg and foot, but I was able to stand. I lost all taste in the right side of my face.

My face on the right side had lost all of its feeling, and I had difficulty swallowing a small sip of water without dribbling. Yes, I could only control the left-hand side of my body. This sucks, as anyone that tries to write with their non-dominant hand; you can see a significant difference in one's abilities (handwriting) when compared to when they do not use their dominant hand.

While lying in bed, I pressed the nurse call button to ask for help, and the nurse who arrived explained again that I had a stroke. The nurse gave me a letter chart and then left. – But I lost the ability to write and spell.

Just like that, my world had changed by an imposed unexpected health issue.

I lay there with my eyes closed, a pillowed on my head to drown out the sounds of the ward, and then I cried. I had hit a new personal low. I reminded myself that I was not dead and pondered what my new life would look like. – I remember the power of purpose, hope and suffering, so I decided to accept my fate/karma and focus on my future and how I rebuild my hope and faith. I remember the advice from my dad, "on any long journey, you need to take small steps."

I understood that suffering was part of life and that it built character. So, I started designing a new dream to give me a new focus and distract me from my problems. I hoped that it would strengthen me in the long term. From my life experience, I understood that real growth happens when you stretch yourself or try something new that makes you comfortable. - The real motivation has to be personal, as this would give me purpose and a target to aim at.

At this stage, I had forgotten the names of everyone I knew, even my two children. However, I knew I loved them and would fight with every ounce of my strength to give them the best life I could manage. Accepting my situation would enable me to move on from where I was.

In the early days after the stroke, I slept between 16 and 20 hours each day and only woke to have a nurse monitor my vitals and remind me to eat.

After three weeks in the hospital, the doctor remarked that I may never speak again.

4. Tiredness

After a brain injury, the brain needs help healing. The reason for tiredness is that the brain needs more energy to process the new demands placed upon it to help recover and the energy required to manage the day-to-day tasks being asked of the body.

(The degree of tiredness can vary from patient to patient, depending on the type of brain injury, the location within the brain injury location, and the patient's health.)

Patients with brain injuries generally suffer from tiredness, which seems never to end. At the start of the stroke, I slept for 18-20 hours a day. Over the subsequent weeks, I slept around 12—15 hours a day. My brain was using all its energy stores to focus on repairing my brain and its pathways. The NHS does not support patients in helping/managing their tiredness...

Table 1: Comparing brain energy between normal and brain injury energy levels - Self-created

Without a Brain Injury	**With** A Brain Injury
In the morning, your battery is full.	In the morning, your battery is partially filled. This is your maximum attainable level.
In the afternoon, energy is used for mental activities, but you still have plenty of energy left.	In the afternoon, after a few mental activities, your battery is almost empty.
In the evening, a substantial part of your energy is used.	In the evening, or sometimes even before, your battery is empty.
At night, your battery is recharged again.	At night, your battery tries to recharge, but it is not strong and cannot be fully recharged.

4.1 Vitamins

Extensive scientific research from Australia supports using vitamins to address tiredness after a brain injury.

In the UK, people with brain injuries are seldom given supplements to address the symptoms of tiredness. I asked the hospital for help with my tiredness, but they offered no options or help to address these symptoms.

Once I was discharged from the hospital, I experimented with different vitamin combinations to determine which daily combinations worked best for me and why.

Vitamin	Pro	Cons
Centrum Advance 50+ (1 tablet daily)	Multi-vitamin. Gives you more than a trace of each vitamin. Help you to replace lost energy.	
Shilajit, seamoss and lions mane (1 tablet only daily)	Helps you think clearer. Reduces brain fog. (Connects your brain pathways) You can buy Shilajit gummies, that are stronger.	Having more tablets each day will make you scratch your head, and your hair will fall out.
Echinacea (1 tablet daily)	This boosts your body's immune system and your ability to fight off cold and flu illnesses.	
Cod olive oil (1 tablet daily)	Lowers your blood pressure and inflammation, is good for your skin, improves eye health, etc	

Table 2: Helpful vitamins - Self-created

The rule with over-using vitamins is that the extra vitamins will be peed out when you go to the toilet.

You should experiment with the combination of vitamins that works best for each individual.

5. Attitude

When you have a significant event that relates to your body, the effects are processed by your mind. Sportspeople often say they must overcome their thoughts/minds before performing at their peak output. Winning the battle of the mind is an essential part of the obstacle as the issue you face. Some say that "controlling your mind" accounts for around 70% of the recovery.

Starting by controlling your mind using the five w's and two h's approach is key to getting your mind ready to receive help:

1. **What** do you focus on?
2. **Why** did you choose this pathway?
3. **Who** helps and who doesn't?
4. **When** do you access it?
5. **Where** do you access it?
6. **How** to help?
7. **How** much?

(I put the above list next to my mirror in my bedroom to remind myself every day that **I can choose to recover** and that **I need to own my recovery**. – When this is listed written out, it acts as a daily reminder that positive change will happen soon.)

For me, the **patient attitude is the most key component of recovery**. Although there have been many times when I felt like giving up, this list kept me focused on my improvement targets and my reasons for success.

Generally, hospital organisation metrics try to help monitor/track service delivery, comprehension of recovery care, and adherence to best practices when managing brain injury patients. However, these metrics are managed by the support person, and measures disappear when the patient is discharged, as hospitals only focus on short-term speech support. - Charities and support groups have finite capital and time to support patients over the long term. The services and standards will be reduced and delivered using a one-size-fits-all approach. This structure and infrastructure delivery problem often frustrates patients, as improvement does not happen linearly.

When researching any change that can affect you, one has to consider the attitude of the people/stakeholders involved. It has been scientifically proven many times in many studies that the difference in people who are successful over-performers when compared to the people who "just turn up" is these two following personal attributes:

1. Have an interest in the subject or area that you focus on. And are willing to stretch/develop their knowledge beyond the topic of study.
2. Attitude to learning (Persistency): to stick to the topic when the topic is complicated or challenging.

Addressing these two factors is key to overcoming most obstacles. (Getting your speech back.)

(Since I won't be allowed to work until my heart doctors give me the green light to return, I have more time to dedicate to improving my skills and knowledge. I use my daily time to work on my speech and comprehension. I know I will never recover fully, but this doesn't stop me from trying to improve myself, one step at a time.)

The attitude to learning is a personal choice and is directly affected by the effort that the patient is willing to invest in their recovery. Put simply, if you put little effort into your recovery, then your recovery will be painful and slow. – You can only improve your outcomes if you put in consistent effort.

Yes, the road to recovery is complicated and very frustrating. When you think you're getting ahead, you have a bad day, and it feels like you're taking two steps back, but you must keep going. If you want to speak again, giving up is not an option.

Around 1 million people each year in the UK and US have stroke/brain injuries. Around 75% of all strokes affect your speech directly. And there is no easy-to-follow, long-term monitoring or treatment for them. Long-term treatment is reserved and accessible for the rich, not everyday people. – This fact bothers me on morale, ethics, and political grounds.

Medical staff and organisations hide behind poorly written instructions that are difficult to follow and hide key information that could otherwise help. These instructions are broken up into many pieces of jargon-orientated information that do not connect the delivery of services to patient or their expectations. In short, the odds of successfully improving your speech and comprehension are stacked against you. – The organisations hide the recovery information by staff and medical staff by confusing you and drip feed just enough information so you will be indebted to the organisation. (I see the organisation's motive is simple; they then charge patients separately for upskilling information to make the patients better.)

After my first stroke, I join I connected with a few stroke groups, and they confirmed that they had similar experiences. I have met many stroke survivors, and many still have little or no long-term help addressing their speech issues or pathways that they can follow to better. I feel like an overlooked social class that has been forgotten on purpose and is being exploited by a raft of medical organisations.

This book is based on the Machiavelli theory, which states, "If you give a man a fish, he can feed himself for a day, but if you teach him to fish, he can feed himself for life." I am opening your eyes to the current tools (which are very poor) and am providing detailed lessons (using an updated Speech framework) that will help you learn to fish again. You can take total ownership of regaining your speech in the long term.

There is no easy way to help you when you have a bad day. I found the following reminders worked for me:

- Remember, other people have it worse than you, and you have no right to complain about life.
- Every new endeavour is challenging initially, but it will become easier if you persevere.

- Every time you think life is dark and tasks are challenging, remind yourself of the positives. For example, I lost all of my film memories in my brain, leaving me with only pictures of my past. Looking back, I see the silver lining: I cannot remember the harm I did to others (if any), so I can choose to live to help others. I now live a happier and more fulfilled life.
- Look out for the silver lining in everything and everyone.
- Look back occasionally to remind yourself how far you have come and praise yourself for this achievement. – Many people have given up long ago when you choose to keep trying.
- Look forward, aim for the stars and dream big. Decide what favour of the power of hope and purpose you have, and I hope you challenge it in a structured and positive way is key.
- Our world comprises rules someone else has created that we must follow. However, we have the right not to agree with these boundaries. If you can, draw the pathways that work for you, and if they don't follow standard conversion, then it is okay. (As long as you don't harm anyone else in your journey.)
- If you can pay forward your happiness by making another person's day, that's great. Helping someone else is great for recharging your soul.
- If this book helps you to help someone else talk again, pass on the information. We owe it to every person to make this world a better place. (I view assisting another person as a good thing.)
- Legacy after a brain injury is complex to envision as you will focus on yourself and not on the world beyond your environment. Make your choices and decisions count, as your options are significantly reduced after a brain injury.

  If you have children, they are your true legacy—not money or tangible items. Children will pass on generational stories to their children, etc.

  (The Chinese say, "nothing dies completely until everything they touch dies." The fact you help another person will live longer than your life or after you die. Your journey to speak again, the skills you have learned, and how you spread the love around you are part of your legacy.)

I like this excerpt from Ernest Hemingway because it helps you understand the patient's mind and needs.

"In our darkest moments, we don't need solutions or advice. What we yearn for is the simple human connection, a quiet presence, a gentle touch. These small gestures are the anchors that hold us steady when life feels too much.

Please don't try to fix me. Don't take on my pain or push away my shadows. Just sit beside me as I work through my inner storms. Be the steady hand I can reach for as I find my way.

My pain is mine to carry, my battles are mine to face. But your presence reminds me that I'm not alone in this vast, sometimes frightening world. It's a quiet reminder that I am worthy of love, even when I feel broken. So, when I lose my way in those dark hours, will you just be here? Not as a rescuer but as a companion. Hold my hand until dawn arrives, helping me remember my strength.

Your silent support is the most precious gift you can give. It's a love that helps me remember who I am, even when I forget."

5.1. Healing from past traumas

To heal from past traumas, you must address the causes and develop your understanding of yourself and your expectations from others. The following table will give you 30 years of psychology research in an easy-to-follow cause-and-effect format that outlines how to heal yourself.:

Table 3: Attitude: Cause and effects – Self-created

Cause	Effects – How to heal.
Anything or any person that angers you	Teaches you forgiveness and compassion for others.
Anything or any person that is frustrating you	Patience with others and yourself.
Anything or any person that has power over you	Teaches you how to get your power back.
Anything or any person that hates you	Teaches you to give unconditional love.
Anything or any person that you fear	Teaches you to have the courage to overcome your fear.
Anything or any person that you can not control	Let them go.
Any person who abandons you	Teach you how to stand up on your own feet.
How a person treats you reflects on your relationship	If the person doesn't put more effort than you, then scale back your effort.

Tip 1

The above list requires you to stop, understand yourself, and build self-awareness. The secret to mastering yourself is understanding your emotional triggers and how they move your thoughts from a dark to a light place. Practice managing your thoughts by categorising your ideas and then rank your thoughts by category. Also, practice counting backwards from five to zero before speaking.

Also, you can practice giving advice back to another person based on another person's attitude. For example, pick a person you respect and ask yourself what advice they would give to someone else instead if the same question were given to them to answer.

6. Stages of Grief

When a person has a brain injury, e.g., a clot-based stroke, they lose a part of their brain function. The area of their brain dies, and the current does not come back to life.

The major event can be looked at as part of their life has died with them, and the patient needs to grieve. - This can be compared to losing a close friend or family member.

The textbook approach for framing grief it is shows that patients will exhibit and encounter the following stages of grief:

1. Denial
2. Anger
3. Bargaining
4. Depression
5. Acceptance

I did not follow the above-prescribed stages of grief. The hospital doctors or nurses could not explain what I would do except.

My journey after my stroke started with depression.

My stages of grief were different than the above-prescribed doctor's stages. In reality, the stages I encountered were:

1. **Depression** - crying and feeling very sorry for myself
2. **Rationality** – Testing and understanding my ability, comparing what I could and could not do well
3. **Fighting for direction, hope, and reasons** — What gave me the most hope was being reminded that "others have it worse than me, and I can live."
4. **Finding purpose**—I found my purpose in wanting to help others speak again and to pass on my knowledge.
5. **Acceptance**—Acceptance came in the form of a change in attitude. Instead of complaining about my disabilities, I started being grateful for the gifts that had been given to me. For

example, previously, I focused on my wants and needs and developed my listening and understanding skills, improving my EQ.

I don't think I have totally accepted my fate, and I do look back fondly on how I was before my stroke, but I focus more often on my gifts and skills than on the items that I have lost. Understand this point, as it is vital. This is the patient's life, and they have to take accountability and believe that they can improve their lives only for themselves and not for anyone else. – Understand that you cannot teach others who don't want to learn.

The best saying I remember when faced with a long, difficult challenge is, " The only way to eat an elephant is one bite at a time."

For people who support people who have suffered brain injury, you will need to be patient with them and ask questions to understand and gauge their state of mind. You can tailor the treatment to suit their needs, wants and attitudes.

7. What are the major types of strokes?

To understand strokes, you must first know that the brain is made of two halves, each holding veins that carry blood around it. Each part of the brain controls a different aspect of a human's actions. Thus, strokes can affect people differently and are very personal; therefore, the symptoms can vary.

A stroke happens when blood flow is disrupted, generally within the brain, and it can lead to cell death and potentially severe neurological (brain) issues. The two main types of strokes happen when:

1. An **ischemic** stroke – Is when the brain has a blood clot, and part of the brain dies
2. A **haemorrhagic** stroke – Is when the brain leaks within itself

When blood from the heart travels to the brain, it first encounters the speech area and our memories. Other symptoms can also affect our physical control, senses, and memory recall. Similar symptoms to those that have Alzheimer's.

The most common symptoms that present after an ischemic stroke are both mental and physical symptoms. The treatments are blood thinners and physical theopathy. The more common symptoms that arise affect the accessing and processing of memories, difficulty in controlling their mouth/speech, swallowing issues, thinking processing issues, and problems coordinating physical movements. It is common for patients to have "brain fog" or the struggle to process their thoughts and physical movements.

For patients that have haemorrhagic stroke, the doctors must first identify where the leak is taking place, and then the doctors must access the brain and stop the leak. This generally involves the patient having some of their head shaved, and an access hatch must be created to access their brain. After the operation, the patients are left with a gruesome scar, a lot of stitches and a lengthy hospital recovery time.

(The best book I found to explain haemorrhagic strokes was "My Stroke of Insight by Jill Bolte Taylor". This is a stroke journal written by a brain surgeon who had a stroke. Understand that haemorrhagic stroke, in the main, does not affect your speech.)

In both types of strokes, patients are left feeling extremely tired and having difficulty processing their brain and physical actions. This tiredness occurs because the brain gathers all the energy available within the body to repair itself.

8. Speech Symptoms

The main speech is classified into Aphasia and Dyspraxia.

I found that when I first lost my speech, I had a blend of both symptoms and over time, my symptoms evolved.

8.1 Aphasia and apraxia

Aphasia and apraxia is caused by damage to the language-dominant side of the brain, usually the left side. It may be brought on by:

- Stroke
- Head injury
- Brain tumour
- Brain infection
- Dementia and/or Alzheimer's disease – both affect the patient's memories

It is unknown whether aphasia causes the complete loss of language structure or problems with accessing and using language.

Key points about aphasia

- Aphasia is a language disorder caused by damage to parts of the brain that control speech and understanding of language.
- Depending on which brain areas are affected, people might have different ability levels to speak, read, write, and understand others.
- Although aphasia might improve over time, many people still experience some loss of language skills. Speech therapy and other tools like computers can help people communicate.

- Aphasia can be difficult and frustrating for both the person with aphasia and family members. It's challenging but essential for family members to be patient and learn the best ways to communicate with their loved ones.

8.2 Dyspraxia

Dyspraxia, or developmental coordination disorder (DCD), is a chronic condition that causes motor (movement) and coordination difficulties.

Signs of dyspraxia include:

- Difficulty organising thoughts and prioritising.
- Difficulty with walking up and down stairs.
- Difficulty with balance — they may bump into objects, fall frequently or seem clumsy.
- Difficulty with sports and activities, such as riding a bike, jumping, catching, and throwing or kicking a ball. They may only participate in activities if they have coordination.
- Difficulty with writing, drawing/colouring and using scissors compared to other children their age.
- Difficulty getting dressed, fastening buttons, brushing their teeth and tying shoelaces.
- Restlessness — limbs may swing or move their arms and legs frequently.

You and your family may become frustrated when trying to perform these tasks.

9. Current Speech Framework

For over 2.5 years, I have struggled to find any information or a framework/guide that could help me understand what has happened to me and the best pathway to follow to help myself or have others teach me to speak again.

The following guide is the only framework available to me:

Figure 1: Psycholinguistic Assessments of Language Processing in Aphasia (1996) by Kay R.Lessers and M.Coltheart

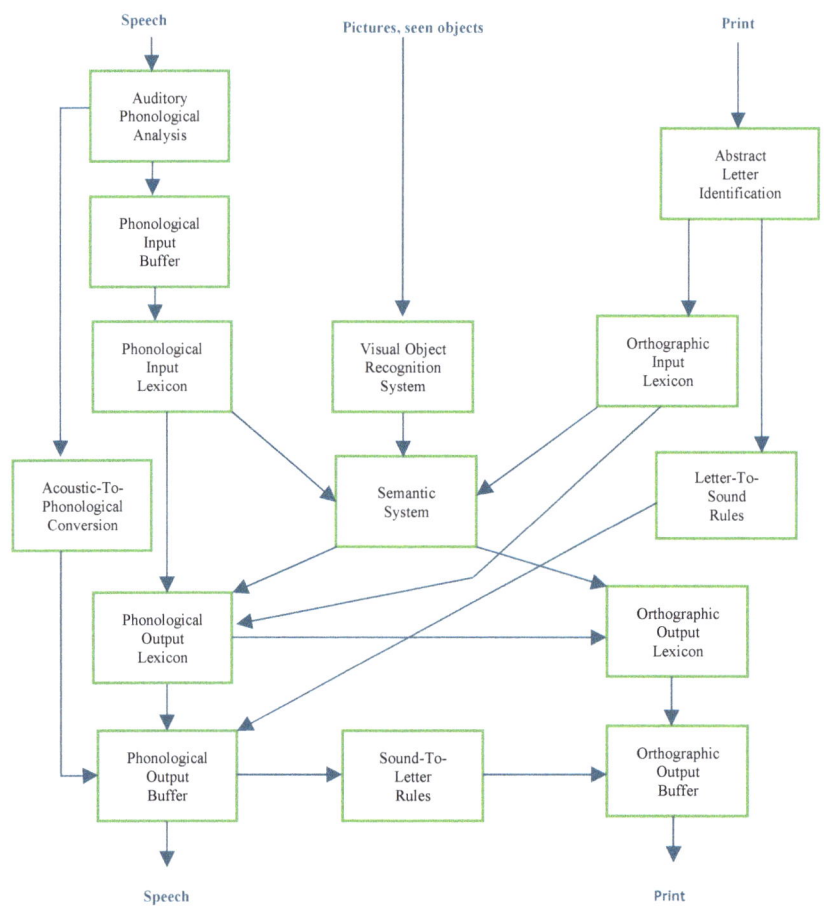

The above framework was written by experienced doctors/researchers who did not explore the subject broadly enough to understand the various end-to-end stages involved in learning to speak again. Consolidating the available past and new global research into one place will centrally organise information and help accelerate the treatments for brain injury survivors who encounter speech issues. This is the point of this book, and I feel duty-bound to pass on my knowledge to others who need it so we can improve the world.

The following noteworthy points can be observed:

- The current framework starts with the patient, assuming that the patient can talk or communicate. - After my stroke, I could not make sounds and had difficulty processing thoughts.
- Processing the brain's thoughts is central to recovery when a brain clot injury occurs. A patient's mental abilities before the stroke are unlearned. (Injuries and recovery pathways are unique to each individual.)
- The phonological (sound/speech) analysis did not happen before the information hit the brain (semantic). – Speech has to be received before it can be analysed.
- Abstract letter identification (print) must happen before the brain can analyse the information. After my stroke, I lost the ability to understand and process letters and numbers.
- The brain processes **stored** speech, pictures, and prints. It then accesses the memories to remap them to fill or build new pathways to the missing information. When a brain injury occurs, one side of the brain is generally affected. The other side works extremely hard to remap the memory to "reinstall" it. The brain is a key facilitator in data handling and processing operations.
- The framework above shows that speech (phonological) only supports the understanding of orthography (pictures) and is not codependent on the other. In the early weeks after my stroke, I could not speak or understand pictures. I lost all memory of films and was left with still pictures of events only.

- The framework shows that sound-to-letter rules depend on phonological input, not the stored semantic system (brain). This suggests that sound-to-letter rules are independent of the brain, which is crazy, as without stored information, we would not be able to understand each other. Moreover, when I lost my speech, I could understand pictures. However, I could not make sounds.

In short, the above framework is mapped for a piece about the speech recovery journey written by people who have not had a general brain clot injury. Additionally, it does not fully map, describe, or understand the end-to-end process for retraining one's mind and speech to recover from a brain injury, and it does not understand the complexities that patients must endure when they recover.

10. Areas of Brain Function

The first step to understanding an injury is understanding how the brain works.

The brain is split into two halves and connected by a tube that shares information between them. The joining halves tubes are similar for males and females; however, the male brain joining tube is narrower than that of the females. – As females' brain joining tubes are wider, they are able to process more information/data at the same time as males.

Two prominent in-and-out veins on each side of the neck feed the brain, the primary nourishment source.

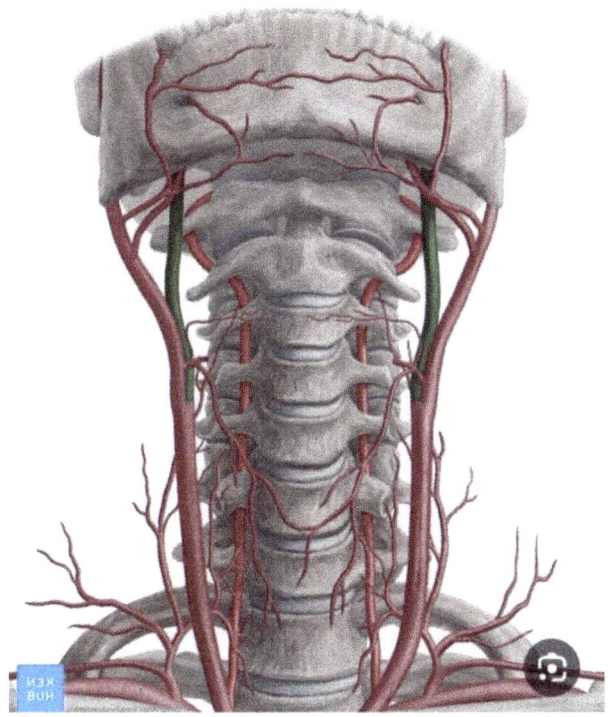

Figure 2: Brain activities areas

The following figure highlights/shows the areas of the brain that control the different aspects of a human being.

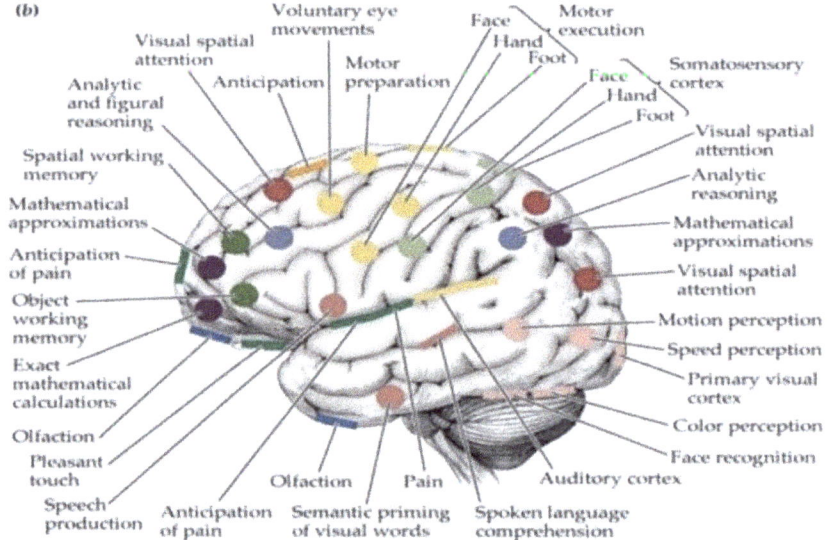

Figure 3: Brain control areas

The veins from the neck merge with the bottom of the brain, and further veins within the brain transfer blood into and out of the brain.

The above figure shows the areas that may be affected by a brain injury. Brain injuries are not the same and affect people differently. The more exercise you can do to retrain your brain, the more likely you will regain its functionality. In short, there are two types of brains: a training brain and an untrained brain.

When I first had my stroke, I lost all my speech and various physical disabilities on my right side, and my memories changed from film to just pictures. At first, after my stroke, I could not remember my own or my children's names. – Don't be hard on yourself; this is when your life is about to change. Over time, you will retain your skills, but it does take time and a lot of dedicated effort.

To retain the brain function, you can use the above figure to focus on the failed areas.

Tip 2

Understanding that the senses feed into and out of the brain is crucial. After a stroke or brain injury, the brain has to work overtime to repair itself and help keep the person alive. When I lost my speech, my senses needed time to recalibrate to help me understand the world around me. I found that when my body could not process thoughts or my speech, I would close my eyes to free up other senses/thinking/brain space to allow me to process other activities, e.g. speaking, thinking, etc. – When I closed my eyes and tried to talk, I could speak with little and on issues.

It is essential to understand that when your senses are recalibrating, your body and mind are in a state of flux, and all the senses are uncontrolled. – It feels similar to watching Superman films, and you see when he was a boy and had to use his senses as he adjusted to being on Earth.

Sitting in a quiet room with your thoughts is the best approach to getting used to the new version of yourself.

Tip 3

A few weeks after my stroke, I could not speak sentences at first, but I could bypass the speaking area of my brain and use the singing area to communicate. I would sing simple words.

Tip 4

Find an experienced chiropractor who can unblock and ease your blood flow in and out of your neck and shoulders. This has been crucial in helping me think more clearly and process information.

Tip 5

When one part of the brain is damaged, the brain on the other side that is unaffected has to remap the thoughts from one side to the other. I found that not all of the words were lost. The words had been moved into a long storage space, and it would take me time to remap each map to the new areas in my mind.

Tip 6

When the brain is affected by injury, the brain has difficulty connecting from one side to another. I experimented with weed to test how the effects could help or hinder my thinking. I found that using CBT has little or no positive impact on my speech, whereas when I used THC, my thinking improved, making the connections with my to improve my thinking and my speech. – Understand that THC is addictive and should be used in controlled environments only.

Don't give up; start with simple words relevant to your life and build from here.

11. Easy Framework: "How to speak again."

The following diagram sets out the framework for "how to speak again after having a brain injury".

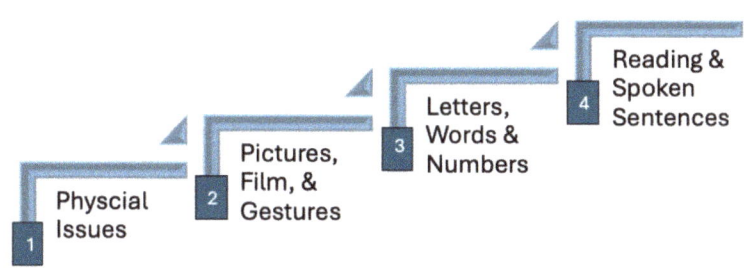

Figure 4: Updated framework on how to speak again
(Source: Self-created)

Figure 4 shows only four steps/stages to improving speech/comprehension.

The recovery journey is shown in steps, which can be tailored to suit the patient's needs.

Different stages can be undertaken simultaneously.

Every stage has a defined set of "abilities" that can be measured and tracked. This allows the patient and the support system to be easily updated, monitored, tracked and shared. Every step allows the patient to build on their comprehension ability.

Record the total at each step/stage; the output gives the sub-Speech Comprehension Index (SCI). Add each sub-SCI level together, and the total SCI can be provided.

11.1 Recording Ability Progress

At every stage, there is a list of abilities that patients have to work on that can be graded from 1 to 5.

Level	Requirement
1	Basic
2	Basic Improver
3	Medium
4	Medium Improver
5	Advance/Fluent

Table 4: Ability Measures (Source: Self-created)

Recording data using the abilities by stage allows you to track the progress of each patient or group. The totals for each stage are added together to give you the overall Speech Comprehension Index.

Firms or patients can store this information to self-manage and track their progress. This information can help doctors, hospitals, and other firms interested in patient outcomes.

(This approach can help organisations to streamline patients' and groups' treatments, therefore improving the targeting of treatments and increasing efficiency within organisations.)

It must be highlighted that the severity of brain injuries and patient attitude will determine the rate of recovery. In some instances, a total recovery may not be possible.

Tip 7

When recording or updating an ability, enter the date the patient achieved the level. This enables patients, support staff, and other organisations to get an overview of the patients in their charge.

12. Stage 1: Physical Issues

When you have a stroke or a brain injury, you lose the ability to control your face and the neck muscles surrounding and within your mouth.

The first stage is the most humbling, as you dibble, cannot make sounds, and cannot be understood by anyone.

The muscles in your mouth and neck do not play nicely with each other. You feel stuck in your mind, but no one can hear you. (It's like being "locked in", but you cannot write, say words, or make sounds.) As a patient, it was the most alone I ever felt.

I craved for someone to take the time to explain what happened to me, but the medical staff ignored me and only approached me when I was given tablets. Never once did the doctors or nurses take the time to explain what happened to me at a pace or in a fashion so I could be understood. In the hospital staff's eyes, I was disabled, and they never looked out for my mental health. I was looked upon as a patient that required "too much attention".

12.1 How to recover?

First, understand that your mouth needs to be divided into four areas: the upper left side, the upper right side, the lower side, and the lower right side.

You will need to exercise each area of the mouth. You can do this by chewing, spitting, swallowing, and making sounds. I found that I could mimic the sounds around me by copying them. Yes, I sounded terrible, but it was necessary.

Tip 8

The following areas will help the patient to recover control of their mouth:

Controlling their swallowing, holding their breath in different parts of the mouth, and their tongue actions. Practice eating using different parts of your mouth to exercise your mouth.

Tip 9

Exercise your mouth and vocal cords: Inflate your cheeks while holding your breath, and then move the air around your mouth (from top to bottom and from side to side). Imagine that you are putting a sweet in your mouth and moving it around.

Tip 10

Begin humming or singing notes. I picked the most straightforward song I knew and repeated it regularly to exercise my vocal cords. – The sound that comes out of your mouth is not as important as the fact that you are trying.

Tip 11

Create a list of simple words the patient and support team can use to encourage them. The words may not make sense to you, but they will help the patient. This is the stage between needing to use a flip book to communicate and moving on to the first/easier words.

12.2 Abilities to track

- Swallowing
- Humming
- Face expressions
- Sounds pitch (Low, medium and high)
- Singing

13. Stage 2: Pictures, Films & Gestures

13.1 Pictures & Films

When I had my first stroke, I could not speak at all, and I was handed a list of the alphabet. But I lost the ability to spell or recognise shapes, which was no help. My world had to be restarted. Letters and pictures looked familiar, but I lost the ability to find the names of people and things and could not organise letters into words or sounds. My short-term and medium memory was trashed. I had to start again from zero.

What helped me start again was that I watched TV to relearn and get familiar with pictures, sounds and letters.

My clever children made me a flip picture book that showed pictures and the words under them. The following words I used frequently:

- Tired
- Sleepy
- Hungary
- Thirsty
- Hot
- Cold
- Family – Brother, sister, children, wife, mum, etc
- Nurse
- Doctor
- Sad
- Wash
- Call

13.2 Gestures

At first, I could only gesture or point at pictures within the flipbook. To communicate my wants and needs, I had to act them out, and I was terrible at acting. My life was pitiful, like a bad game of charades. The right side of my body was not working well, and I could only point (using my left hand) to pictures.

When I looked at or heard the TV, my mind was relearning the sounds and words that I had forgotten. Over time, my children and I added new words to the list, which helped me develop my lexicon and relationships with my friends, family, and the wider world.

Tip 12

When you watch TV, switch on the subtitles. This helps your mind connect sounds with letters and your memory. You can enhance your memory recall by remapping your sounds with your mind.

For me and other stroke survivors, our memory has not lost words; instead, it has stored memories in long-term memory. It takes time to remap the brain/mind from one side to the other and re-access memories.

It took me 4-8 times to remember or access the pictures, films, and memories. You have to be very patient at the start, as this is the start of the journey. You will get super tired, as your brain needs time to recover from the new stress (remapping your thoughts, learning sounds and words you had forgotten). I found that at the beginning, I could only be awake for 10-15 minutes before I fell asleep.

13.3 Abilities to track

- Understanding pictures, films and gestures
- Track the patient's ability to communicate using their dominant hand.

14. Stage 3: Letters, Words, & Numbers

14.1 Letters

Understanding letters is the first step to communicating. You must list all the letters of the alphabet and practice saying the sounds of each letter, one at a time.

(Practice saying letters is the perfect way to exercise the mouth and connect it with the sounds in the brain.)

When you have mastered the basic letter sounds, then you can practice the following complex speed sounds: (Know that some of the sounds are silent when written or spoken.)

Complex Speed Sounds

Consonant sounds

f	l	m	n	r	s	v	z	sh	th	ng
ff	ll	mm	nn	rr	ss	ve	zz	ti		nk
ph	le	mb	kn	wr	se		s	ci		
			gn		c		se			
					ce					

b	c	d	g	h	j	p	qu	t	w	x	y	ch
bb	k	dd	gg		g	pp		tt	wh			tch
	ck		gu		ge							
	ch				dge							

Vowel sounds

a	e	i	o	u	ay	ee	igh	ow
	ea				a-e	e-e	i-e	o-e
					ai	y	ie	oa
					a	ea	i	o
						e	y	oe

oo	oo	ar	or	air	ir	ou	oy	ire	ear	ure
u-e			oor	are	ur	ow	oi			
ue			ore		er					
ew			aw							
			au							

Table 5: Complex Letter Speed Sounds

14.2 Letter & Words

When you start practising, you begin with words that start with M, P, B, and W and then move on to the vowels. - The suggested words are listed to target the different areas within the mouth and by the level of difficulty. The more symbols in a word, the harder it is to say.

Table 6: Words to learn/practice first

M	Level 1 - Monosyllabic	Level 2	Level 3 – Multisyllabic
1	Meat	Mitten	Mechanical
2	Must	Machine	Monotonous
3	Main	Major	Manufacture
4	Mat	Measure	Musical
5	Might	Mixture	Macaroni
6	March	Magic	Motivation
7	Map	Metal	Mandatory
8	Mouth	Midnight	Municipality
9	Mum	Mister	Meteorology
10	Mould	Member	Machinery
11	Mad	Meter	Millennium
12	Mere	Mother	Multiplication
13	Mix	Muddy	Memorial
14	Musk	Memo	Mysterious
15	Make	Manner	Magnificent
16	Mail	Mermaid	Medication
17	More	Minute	Mathematics
18	Men	Monday	Melancholy
19	Month	Mustache	Military
20	May	Mental	Miscellaneous

P	Level 1 - Monosyllabic	Level 2	Level 3 – Multisyllabic
1	Pour	Paper	Pyjamas
2	Page	Poodle	Publication
3	Peel	Puppet	Potato
4	Pole	Puzzle	Peppermint
5	Par	Panel	Pavilion
6	Pond	Pepper	Pentagon
7	Pure	Parole	Pedestrian
8	Peach	Posture	Popular
9	Peer	Peasant	Purposeful
10	Pull	Patties	Pacific
11	Pair	Paddle	Pathetic
12	Pit	Pencil	Perceptible
13	Park	Pimple	Particular
14	Paste	People	Palomino
15	Pen	Payment	Potential
16	Porch	Package	Paediatrician
17	Pain	Parrot	Partnership
18	Pace	Pupil	Perfectionist
19	Paid	Police	Paragraph
20	Patch	Pamphlet	Possession

B	Level 1 - Monosyllabic	Level 2	Level 3 – Multisyllabic
1	Born	Below	Binoculars
2	Bag	Bumper	Balcony
3	Barn	Bowling	Barbarian
4	Bug	Boston	Bacteria
5	Bull	Bother	Benefit
6	Bite	Beaver	Biography
7	Boy	Banner	Bureaucracy
8	Bat	Burning	Barracuda
9	Beast	Bitter	Bipartisan
10	Beg	Believe	Benediction
11	Big	Business	Bonanza
12	Bone	Basement	Badminton
13	Bus	Basket	Belligerent
14	Boast	Batter	Basketball
15	Beef	Birthday	Bibliography
16	Best	Billion	Begonia
17	Bun	Better	Behaviour
18	Bank	Bases	Beverage
19	Ball	Berry	Bilateral
20	Bend	Balloon	Beneficial

W	Level 1 - Monosyllabic	Level 2	Level 3 – Multisyllabic
1	Wife	Wagon	Wonderful
2	Win	Water	Wilderness
3	Waste	Welcome	Witticism
4	Wick	Wire	Wintergreen
5	Wall	Western	Watermelon
6	Warm	Weapon	Woodpecker
7	Wood	Workbook	Wastebasket
8	Week	Wallet	Wallpaper
9	Want	Woman	Waterproof
10	Work	Weather	Washable
11	Watch	Without	Willingly
12	Wipe	Wander	Winterise
13	Went	Waffle	Warranty
14	Wing	Wicker	Windowpane
15	Word	Warning	Wizardry
16	Wide	Wednesday	Wistfulness
17	Wage	Wisdom	Windbreaker
18	Were	Walnut	Wallaby
19	Wake	Wicked	Westerly
20	Weed	Waver	Winterise

Table 7: Vowels

Ei/A	Level 1 - Monosyllabic	Level 2	Level 3 – Multisyllabic
1	Ape	Able	Aorta
2	Aim	Acorn	Apiary
3	Ache	Acre	Aqueous
4	Aid	Apex	Apricot
5	Ail	April	Abraham
6	Age	Amen	Aimlessness
7	Ate	Aching	Asymmetric
8	Abe	Aphid	Asymptomatic
9	Ace	Agent	Anciently
10	Aides	Amos	Asocial

Ae/A	Level 1 - Monosyllabic	Level 2	Level 3 – Multisyllabic
1	Add	Adam	Advantageous
2	Act	Action	Academic
3	Am	Adder	Agony
4	At	Axel	Accurate
5	As	Ashes	Analyse
6	Axe	Acid	Attitude
7	Aft	Asset	Abstraction
8	Ash	Accent	Agitation
9	Apt	Anger	Accelerate
10	Asp	Admit	Ambidextrous

I/E	Level 1 - Monosyllabic	Level 2	Level 3 – Multisyllabic
1	Each	Eager	Easy-going
2	Ear	Eagle	Eavesdropping
3	Ease	Easel	Eager beaver
4	Eat	Easement	Eagle-eyed
5	East	Eject	Equalise
6	Eaves	Eastern	Ecology
7	Eel	Easy	Ethology
8	Eared	Eavesdrop	Equilibrium
9	Eased	Either	Easiest
10	Eats	Earache	Ear-splitting

E/E	Level 1 - Monosyllabic	Level 2	Level 3 – Multisyllabic
1	Egg	Echo	Everyone
2	Ebb	Ember	Ebony
3	Edge	Edges	Episode
4	Elk	Ever	Economical
5	Ed	Epic	Editor
6	Etch	Emblem	Emperor
7	End	Elder	Emily
8	Elf	Embrace	Edification
9	Else	Essay	Ecstatic
10	Elm	Edit	Educator

Ai/I	Level 1 - Monosyllabic	Level 2	Level 3 – Multisyllabic
1	Eye	Idea	Identical
2	Ice	Ion	Itinerary
3	I'd	Irate	Ivory
4	Ike	Irish	Isolation
5	Ides	Iron	Idolatry
6	Ayes	Ivy	Idealistically
7	I'm	Island	Icicle
8	Iced	Icy	Iodine
9	Ike's	Idol	Ideology
10	Eyed	Ideal	Irony

I/I	Level 1 - Monosyllabic	Level 2	Level 3 – Multisyllabic
1	It	Impress	Individual
2	In	Igloo	Imitation
3	Is	Income	Inconsequential
4	Ink	Itself	International
5	If	Invent	Ingenious
6	Ill	Ignore	Illegal
7	Imp	Infant	Impatient
8	Inch	Improve	Initial
9	Itch	Ill-bred	Irregular
10	It's	Insect	Ingredient

O/O	Level 1 - Monosyllabic	Level 2	Level 3 – Multisyllabic
1	Oath	Opal	Omission
2	Owe	Open	Ownership
3	Oaf	Okay	Ohio
4	Oak	Owner	Omega
5	Ode	Opaque	Olympic
6	Own	Omit	Oceanography
7	Oat	Ogre	Omaha
8	Oh	Omen	Overture
9	Owed	Ozone	Opening
10	Old	Ocean	Opacity

A/O	Level 1 - Monosyllabic	Level 2	Level 3 – Multisyllabic
1	Odds	Obsess	Occupation
2	Odd	Oxtail	Opposite
3	On	Oddball	Obsolete
4	Os	Onset	Ottawa
5	Ow	Oblong	October
6	Oi	Oxford	Objection
7	Ox	Omelette	Optimistic
8	Ops	Occult	Oxidize
9	Opt	Oddest	Observer
10	Oft	Oxen	Oddity

U/U	Level 1 - Monosyllabic	Level 2	Level 3 – Multisyllabic
1	You	Usage	Ukulele
2	Your	Youthful	Utility
3	Youth	User	Unicycle
4	Use	Usurp	Utopian
5	You'll	Union	Utensil
6	Youths	Unit	Utilitarian
7	Yule	Yukon	Ukrainian
8	You'd	Useful	Unanimous
9	You've	Yuletide	Uniform
10	Yew	Unite	Unilateral

U/U	Level 1 - Monosyllabic	Level 2	Level 3 – Multisyllabic
1	Ugh	Umpire	Umbrella
2	Ump	Uncle	Unbelievable
3	Urn	Ugly	Undergraduate
4	Us	Under	Uneasy
5	Up	Utmost	Upheaval
6	Umps	Usher	Ugly-duckling
7	Urns	Until	Uppity
8	Umped	Umpteen	Umbilical
9	Um	Upset	Uncertainty
10	Ups	Unborn	Unforgettable

OU	Level 1 - Monosyllabic	Level 2	Level 3 – Multisyllabic
1	Ouch	Owls	Outrageous
2	Out	Outage	Outermost
3	Owl	Ounces	Owlishly
4	Oust	Owlish	Outboard motor
5	Ounce	Ousted	Owlishness
6	Our	Ourselves	Outmanoeuvred
7	Ousts	Owlet	Outspoken
8	Ours	Outlaw	Outnumber
9	Outs	Outback	Out bargain
10	Oud	Outdoor	Outgoing

Ae+R	Level 1 - Monosyllabic	Level 2	Level 3 – Multisyllabic
1	Air	Aerate	Aerator
2	Ere	Airedale	Aerobatics
3	Aired	Airborne	Aerodynamics
4	Heir	Airy	Aerosol
5	Airs	Airplane	Airliner
6	Heirs	Ergo	Air conditioner
7		Airflow	Air mattress
8		Airport	Air sickness
9		Air head	Aeronautics
10		Airmail	Agronomic

AW	Level 1 - Monosyllabic	Level 2	Level 3 – Multisyllabic
1	Ought	Offer	Automatic
2	Off	Author	Auspicious
3	Or	Often	Audiologist
4	Orb	Awful	Automobile
5	Oar	Awkward	Audience
6	Auld	Office	Awesome
7	Awl	Offhand	Officer
8	Awe	Offered	Awkwardness
9	Awed	Offers	Audible
10	Awes	Authored	Auditory

A	Level 1 - Monosyllabic	Level 2	Level 3 – Multisyllabic
1		Achieve	Abandon
2		Adore	Accumulation
3		Adopt	American
4		Agree	Abolish
5		Abyss	Analogy
6		Account	Agreeable
7		Attempt	Analogy
8		Amount	Apologise
9		Asleep	Association
10		Awhile	Adoring

Tip 13

At Levels 2 and 3, I split and broke the words into sounds to make them. Marking or underlining the sounds helped me relearn the words.

Tip 14

Practice putting the words into sentences and into tongue twisters.

Tip 15

Take your time when sounding out the letter in the word. I found that using a phonic dictionary to check words I struggled with.

I found that using the Google Translate program (a free app), you can look up words and get help with their spelling. The apps also allow you to hear the sounds that make up the word and see its phonic spelling.

Tip 16

I practised singing songs, combining my talking and speech abilities. By singing, you bypass the areas of the brain that manage your speech.

(FYI - I only sing behind a closed and locked door because my voice is that flat..)

14.3 Numbers

There is no shortcut to learning numbers. The easy way to learn numbers is to write each number up to 100 and then say each number out loud again and again until you remember the numbers.

You must also learn to write each number in longhand, e.g. one, two, three, etc.

Once you have mastered the numbers up to 100, you can build the units: thousands, tens of thousands, millions, etc.

This will give you a basis upon which to build your number knowledge.

Once you have learned your numbers, you must learn how to apply the numbers by using essential functions: adding, taking away, dividing, and multiplying.

Tip 17

I started with dice (numbers up to 6 only), then used cards (which require counting up to 15) and played checkers.

To learn simple maths functions, I downloaded a free app called Cross Maths from the Apple App Store. The app allows you to practice and relearn how to apply math functions, and you can select the skill level that applies to you.

13.2 Abilities to track

- Track the words you can say (fluently), what you cannot and what is difficult. – This will help you and your support/nurse to focus on the help areas that apply to you.
- Track when the patient can build on the words by applying the words to sentences.
- Track when the patient can use the words to make tongue twisters.
- Track the numbers that you can say and what is more challenging.
- Track the number level that the patient can remember.
- Test the patient with numbers by asking them to recall numbers that increased and decreased in value.
- Test the patient with basic mathematical functions.

15. Stage 4: Reading & Spoken

To test the survivor's spoken word, I suggest the following tests to gauge/monitor mental, sensory and speech ability.

Tests 1-4

1/ Gestures to spoken ability:

Measure the accuracy

Mental processing speed

Speed of delivery

2/ Pictures to spoken ability:

Measure the accuracy,

Mental processing speed

Speed of delivery

3/ Film to spoken ability:

Measure the accuracy,

Mental processing speed

Speed of delivery

4/ Creative speech ability

Record and monitor the patient's ability to speak creatively with open and closed eyes.

Each of the four tests will guide the support person in identifying the areas in the brain that they need to target to help the patient relearn or map new connections within the brain attributed to each sense-processing activity.

Tip 18

The patient can improve their communication ability by slowing down their thinking, varying the speed of delivery, and minimising sensory overloading.

Tip 19

When you start reading again, I suggest reading children's books that use simple words. As you practice, you will improve your spoken words, breath control, and mouth muscles.

When reading and speaking words or sentences, you must develop your voice to include emotions, which brings life to your speech.

The following table will guide you on how to develop your reading and speaking skills to add emotions:

Table 8: Guide to Adding Emotions to Speech – Self-created

Voice	Guide	Comments
Volume	Loud	Sodcasting – Being loud
Volume	Quiet	Whispering: secrets, soft voice to share info helps the listener to focus on the content of the message.
Register	Where our sounds come from: nose (high-pitched), throat (where the sound comes from), and diagram (depth).	Varying the source of sounds can change the level of trust of the received.
Timbre	People prefer warm and rich sounds.	Managing yourself: breathing has an effect on your sounds, and changing your posture (standing or sitting).
Pace	Talking quickly implies that you are excited, and think that slow talking is boring and shows that you are struggling to talk.	Slow your speech, as it will enable you to process your thoughts more easily.
Prosody	This is the up and down or singing of voice when talking.	People that talk in a flat way are hard to understand (monotony).
Silence	Good to help the listener process the info/message.	Don't need to fill silence with noise.

You will experience difficulty sorting and grouping thoughts into categories as you rebuild your lexicon.

Tip 20

While reading the text, I suggest you imagine you are an actor giving a speech.

You can liven up your voice by pretending to be a famous person you can imitate. Please enjoy this stage and remember how far you have come in your recovery. My children love to laugh at me when I make mistakes, reminding me of when I used to read books to them as children before settling them down to bed. Yes, I did the silly voices.

Speaking is one aspect of language, as is listening to the words, so keep this in mind when speaking.

Tip 21

Encourage the patients to imagine themselves in a shop and ask them to describe what they see. Then, repeat this exercise in other environments, such as the gym, garage, airport, recovery groups, or hospital.

15.1 Abilities to track

- Track how the patient processed their thoughts and senses into speech.
- Track how creativity is applied in spoken words, eyes open/closed.
- Track how the patients can develop their speaking skills in the above areas: Volume, register, timbre, pace, prosody, and silence.
- Test the patient to speak by reading out a book to an audience.
- Test how the patients can group or categorise their thoughts and speech when discussing different topics and environments.
- Test how memory recall works with eyes closed and opened.

16. Useful apps

To help you develop your mind and abilities, I listed the major apps that helped me regain my speech and improve my comprehension.

Table 9: Speech Apps Used – Self-created

Name	Cost	Reason	
		Positive	**Negative**
Advance Language	30days free	Lots of games to help you test and re-learn memory skills.	Does not give an example of how to speak again.
Cody Cross	Free	A memory test that your general knowledge. Tests your spelling.	Some of the words are American, so expect a lot of z instead of s.
Cross Math	Free	Great app that helps you relearn how to process basic maths functions. You can vary the skill levels.	
Cue Speak	30days free	Give you lots of games/examples of how to speak again. You can slow down the speech of the examples you see. You have a person that shows you how to say words that you can copy.	Does not give you the phonic spelling of words, so silent letters, etc, are hard to copy
Google Translate	Free	Enables you to type the words and correct your spelling as you write. Hear the words, and also you will see the phonic spelling of words, so you can pronounce the words correctly.	
Grammarly	Vary	Helps you to spell and write in a concise way.	

		It helps you to simplify and adjust the tone of your writing.	
Mahjong	Free	Helps with your memory, recall, positioning, etc. – this is an advance recovery app.	Some of the tiles can be hard to understand and match.
Scattergorires	Free	Good for developing the categories of objects and names.	
Solitaire	Free	Good to learn how to count again.	
Spot the Difference	Free	Developing your space awareness.	
Sudoku	Free	Test your space awareness. Test your ability to use numbers.	
Syn-Ant	Free	The words are timed and not easy to follow.	Many of the words are very odd, and it is difficult to see their relationships.

17. How to Improve Comprehension

Improving comprehension involves a mix of strategies that can enhance your understanding of texts, whether you're reading for school, work, or pleasure. Here are some practical tips:

1. **Preview the Material**: Before diving in, skim the headings, subheadings, and any summaries or questions. This will give you a framework for what to expect.

2. **Active Reading**: Engage with the text by highlighting key points, taking notes, or asking questions as you read. This keeps your mind focused.

3. **Summarise**: After reading a section, pause to summarise what you've just read in your own words. This reinforces understanding.

4. **Ask Questions**: As you read, ask yourself questions about the material. What is the main idea? How does this connect to what I already know?

5. **Read Aloud**: Hearing the words can help reinforce understanding, especially for complex or dense texts.

6. **Practice Active Recall**: Test yourself on the material without looking at the text. This helps strengthen memory and comprehension.

7. **Discussion**: Talk about what you've read with others. Explaining concepts to someone else can deepen your understanding.

8. **Slow Down**: If you're having trouble comprehending, slow your pace. Taking time to absorb information can be more beneficial than rushing through it.

9. **Regular Practice**: Like any skill, comprehension improves with practice. Read a variety of texts regularly to build your skills.

10. **Speaking**: Vocalise your day-to-day activities, as this helps you reconnect or remap the missing links between one side of the brain and the other.

Implementing these strategies gradually can lead to noticeable improvements in your comprehension abilities!

Tip 22

To rebuild the thought categories in your brain again, encourage the patients to imagine they are in a shop and ask them to describe what they see. Then, repeat this exercise in other environments, e.g., the gym, garage, airport, recovery groups, hospital, etc. – This is very helpful for stroke and Alzheimer patients.

I found playing a game called Scattergories very beneficial in helping with day-to-day memory recall as it helps you categorise and order your thoughts.

18. Tracking Speech & Comprehension

Monitoring and tracking comprehension is essential for patient improvement.

Table 10: Tracking Speech Comprehension Performance – Self-created

Comprehension Activities	Beginner		Immediate		Fluent
Stage 1: Physical Issues	1	2	3	4	5
Swallowing					
Humming					
Face expressions					
Sounds pitch (Low, medium and high)					
Singing					

Stage 2: Picture, Films & Gestures

Understanding pictures, films and gestures					
Track the patient's ability to communicate using their dominant hand.					

Stage 3: Letters, Words & Numbers

Track the words you can say (fluently), what you cannot and what is difficult. – This will help you and your support/nurse to focus on the help areas that apply to you.					
Track when the patient can build on the words by applying the words to sentences.					

Track when the patient can use the words to make tongue twisters.					
Track the numbers that you can say and what is more challenging.					
Track the number level that the patient can remember.					
Test the patient with numbers by asking them to recall numbers that increased and decreased in value.					
Test the patient with basic mathematic functions.					

Stage 4: Reading & Spoken

Test 1 (Gestures): Measure of accuracy					
Test 1 (Gestures): Mental processing speed					
Test 1 (Gestures): Speed of delivery					
Test 2 (Pictures): Measure of accuracy					
Test 2 (Pictures): Mental processing speed					
Test 2 (Pictures): Speed of delivery					
Test 3 (Film): Measure of accuracy					
Test 3 (Film): Mental processing speed					
Test 3 (Film): Speed of delivery					
Test 4: Creative speaking with eyes **open**					
Test 4: Creative speaking with eyes **closed**					
Track how the patients can develop their speaking skills:					
Volume – Loud and quiet					
Register – Nose (high), throat or diaphragm (depth)					

Tibre – Position (Standing or sitting)				
Pace – Talking fast shows excitement. Slow is bored or struggling				
Prosody – The up or down of talking				
Silence – Appreciate the silence in between topics				
Test the patient to speak by reading out a book to an audience.				
Test how the patients can group or categorise their thoughts and speech when discussing different topics and environments.				
Test how memory recall works with eyes closed and opened.				

Use Table (10) to track the speech and monitor the patient's progress.

17.1 How to use the table

1. Measure the patient's baseline or starting point by going through each stage and each skill by entering the date the patient was examined and/or when they achieved (date) their skill level/milestone.
2. In each box, record the date the patient's comprehension ability increased. Each ability can be tracked individually.
3. Total each ability by step; then, you will have the total by each step.
4. Totalled up to give each Speech patient's speech Comprehension level/Index (SCI).

(The four stages and the primary "skill" items are listed that helped the support staff and you track your speech development. The skill list gives an overview of the primary skill items that you need to achieve. - The list of skills can be added to and further developed to suit your patient's and practice requirements.)

Tip 23

Patient support can periodically re-test the patient to track the development of the support staff and organisations that have been delivered. By updating the abilities and, in turn, the Speech Index, you can identify the areas to focus on with each patient. This approach can also help the support staff/organisation monitor the delivery performance of services and their effect on their patients.

19. Overview of Comprehension

I found the most straightforward way to get an overview of the patients' skills/abilities and group targets is to present the information in a pictural (chart-radar) format and suggest the following approach:

Figure 5: Suggested pictorial tracking methods using the radar charting method – Self-created

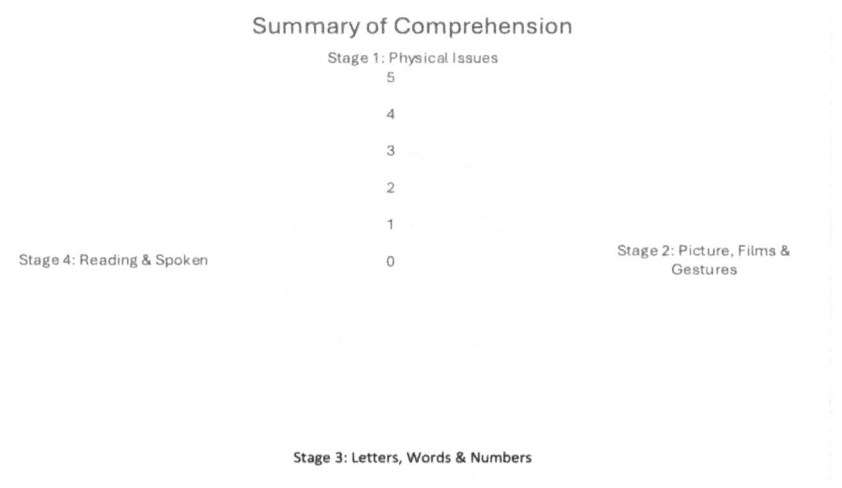

Following the four steps allows for a multi-level engagement with each stakeholder group engaged in service delivery.

This radar charting format allows the medical/support staff to get an overview of each patient's needs quickly and, in a structured, staged way, determine where to focus their efforts on an individual, teaching, group, or organisational level.

When support groups vary with patients with varying needs, organisations can adapt their practices to allow the groups to be split into smaller/sub-groups with similar needs. This is a more cost-efficient delivery of services, improves care targeting towards patients, and, more importantly, this approach can speed up and shorten the patient's recovery time.

Tip 24

Organisations will get a total overview of SCI for each stage. This can help group organisers run cost-efficient focus groups that appeal to patients with similar symptoms. Splitting groups into development stages allows you to deliver/service more patients simultaneously. Patients will readily accept help if they understand and relate to patients with similar speech issues. The journey of regaining one's speech is personal, as is the Speech or Comprehension Index.

The Speech Comprehension Index/SCI can then be compared by patient stage, group, and support staff skill level, and the organisation's recovery rate can provide a simple overview of progress. This simplified approach can help with patient grouping, resource assignment and allocation, and patient processing management.

20. Effects of CBD and THC

Different countries have different views and regulations towards the use of THC and CBD.

As with many brain injury patients that I have engaged with online stroke groups and in person, there is a strong agreement that taking THC can be beneficial to opening the mind/neuro pathways and helping the patients with their recovery.

In desperation to help myself and others shorten the mind recovery process, I explored the effects of THC and CBD.

The mechanisms to take the drug can vary: smoking, vapes, food, gummies, etc.

20.1 CBD

I found CBD was a good alternative to taking painkillers, and I did not have any noticeable side effects.

CBD did not help with the mind recovery.

21.2 THC

I found that THC was very effective at opening the pathways in my mind. The pathways connecting my mind and my speech improved noticeably. I could think more clearly and creatively, and my speech also improved.

When using THC and closing my eyes to practise speaking, my memory and speech improved significantly. My mind (speech, memory recall, synchronisation of word use) felt enhanced on many levels. However, I found that the effects of THC were short-lived, providing only temporary help and relief.

After the effects wore off, my speech returned to a lower level than I started. It was as though the boost I had drained my energy, and my thinking slowed for a day or so after taking THC.

THC helped increase my creativity (creating new pathways in the brain), confidence, memory recall, and other valuable areas that boost my brain and physical recovery. Once developed, these abilities would stay developed.

THC is addictive and should be used carefully. – It can give the patient the munchies and can affect your weight.

Tip 25

If you take THC, make a list of tasks that you want to focus on, such as practising learning hard-to-say words, sentences, or phases. You will notice a direct improvement in the patient's speech.

I practise singing songs, combining my talking and speech abilities. By singing, you bypass the areas of the brain that manage your speech.

(FYI - I only sing behind a closed and locked door because my voice is that flat. To protect others...)

21. Organisational Support/tools

The following general hospital organisation metrics help ensure high-quality comprehension recovery care and adherence to best practices when managing brain injury patients. However, these metrics and standards disappear when the patient is discharged. Charities and support groups have finite capital to support patients over the long term, and many services and standards will be reduced.

Tracking the Speech Comprehension Index is a simple way to create a record that can follow the patient's recovery journey.

- Better tracking of patients and their performance allows organisations to monitor their patients, staff, and management and draw data (patterns) from the results.

21.1 Infrastructure Performance Guide

Hospitals use a variety of metrics to monitor performance, including:

1. **Patient Outcomes**: Measures like mortality rates, readmission rates, and complication rates help assess the effectiveness of care.

2. **Patient Satisfaction**: Surveys and feedback tools, such as the HCAHPS (Hospital Consumer Assessment of Healthcare Providers and Systems) survey, gauge patient experiences.

3. **Operational Efficiency**: Metrics such as average length of stay, bed occupancy rates, and patient throughput provide insights into the efficiency of hospital operations.

4. **Financial Performance**: Key financial indicators include revenue cycle metrics, cost per patient, and profit margins.

5. **Clinical Quality Indicators** include adherence to evidence-based clinical guidelines and protocols for specific conditions (e.g., surgical site infections and sepsis management).

6. **Staffing Metrics**: Ratios of staff to patients, staff turnover rates, and employee satisfaction scores help evaluate workforce effectiveness.

7. **Access to Care**: Wait times for appointments, emergency department wait times, and the number of patients seen can indicate accessibility.

8. **Safety Metrics**: Tracking incidents of adverse events, medication errors, and patient falls helps ensure a safe environment.

9. **Compliance and Accreditation**: Meeting standards set by organisations like The Joint Commission or CMS, including tracking compliance with regulations.

10. **Population Health Metrics**: Monitoring metrics related to community health, such as disease prevalence and vaccination rates, can help hospitals assess their broader impact.

These metrics provide a comprehensive view of a hospital's performance and guide quality, safety, and patient care improvements.

21.2 Nurse Performance Measurement

Hospitals measure nurse performance in treating stroke patients using several key metrics, including:

1. **Time to Treatment**: Tracking how quickly nurses administer critical interventions, such as thrombolysis (e.g., tPA), after a stroke is diagnosed.

2. **Adherence to Protocols**: Measuring compliance with established stroke care protocols and guidelines, such as the American Heart Association/American Stroke Association recommendations.

3. **Patient Assessment Accuracy**: Evaluating the effectiveness of nurses in conducting initial stroke assessments, including the use of the NIHSS.

4. **Patient Monitoring**: Assessing how well nurses monitor vital signs and neurological status post-stroke to identify complications early.

5. **Medication Administration**: Tracking adherence to medication protocols, including timely administration of anticoagulants or antiplatelet agents.

6. **Patient Education**: Evaluating nurses' effectiveness in educating patients and families about stroke, recovery, and prevention strategies.

7. **Documentation Quality**: Assessing the completeness and accuracy of nursing documentation related to stroke care and patient progress.

8. **Patient Outcomes**: Monitoring outcomes such as improvements in mobility, speech, and functional independence, as well as readmission rates.

9. **Patient Satisfaction**: Gathering feedback on patients' and families' perceptions of nursing care through surveys or direct interviews.

10. **Continuing Education and Training**: Tracking participation in ongoing education related to stroke care and best practices.

21.3 Stroke metrics to monitor the recovery of patients

Hospitals use several specific metrics to monitor the recovery of stroke survivors, including:

1. **Functional Independence Measure (FIM)**: Assesses a patient's level of disability and functional independence after a stroke.

2. **Modified Rankin Scale (MRS)**: A standard measure for assessing the degree of disability or dependence in daily activities.

3. **National Institutes of Health Stroke Scale (NIHSS)**: This scale evaluates the severity of a stroke and tracks changes in neurological function during recovery.

4. **Barthel Index**: This index measures a patient's ability to perform basic activities of daily living (ADLs) and helps assess recovery progress.

5. **Quality of Life Assessments**: Surveys, such as the Stroke Impact Scale (SIS), evaluate health-related quality of life from the patient's perspective.

6. **Rehabilitation Progress**: Monitoring specific rehabilitation goals, such as improvements in mobility, speech, and swallowing.

7. **Readmission Rates**: Tracking the frequency of readmissions for stroke-related complications or secondary strokes.

8. **Time to Rehabilitation**: Measures the time from stroke onset to the initiation of rehabilitation services.

9. **Medication Adherence**: Evaluating adherence to prescribed post-stroke medications to prevent recurrence and complications.

10. **Psychosocial Assessments**: Monitoring for depression and anxiety, which are common after strokes, using standardised screening tools.

These metrics help healthcare providers tailor recovery plans, assess the effectiveness of interventions, and improve overall care for stroke survivors.

22. Creating Analysis to Measure Performance & Quality

The following are analysis tools that any health organisation can use to measure their services' quality and performance.

22.1 Diagnostic analysis

Diagnostic analysis involves examining data to identify the causes of problems or trends. Here are some examples of approaches used in diagnostic analysis:

1. **Root Cause Analysis (RCA)**: (Six Sigma approach is required)
   - **Example**: If hospital falls increase, RCA may be employed to investigate underlying causes, such as inadequate staff training, poor environmental design, or patient mobility issues.

2. **Regression Analysis**:
   - **Example**: A healthcare organisation might use regression analysis to understand the relationship between staffing levels and patient outcomes, identifying how changes in nurse-to-patient ratios affect readmission rates.

3. **Benchmarking**:
   - **Example**: A hospital compares its infection rates to those of similar institutions to identify areas needing improvement and analyse discrepancies to determine best practices.

4. **Trend Analysis**:
   - **Example**: Analysing patient satisfaction scores over time to detect patterns, such as seasonal fluctuations, and understanding factors contributing to these changes.

5. **Variance Analysis**:
   - **Example**: Review budget variances to determine why actual department costs differ from budgeted figures. This may involve examining staffing, equipment usage, or supply costs.

6. **Flowcharting**:
   - **Example**: Creating a flowchart of patient discharge processes to identify bottlenecks or delays that may contribute to extended hospital stays.

7. **Fishbone Diagram (Ishikawa)**:
   - **Example**: A multidisciplinary team uses a fishbone diagram to categorise potential causes of medication errors, including factors related to people, processes, and equipment.

8. **SWOT Analysis**:
   - **Example**: A healthcare facility conducts a SWOT analysis to identify internal strengths and weaknesses and external opportunities and threats related to its stroke care program.

9. **Qualitative Analysis**:
   - **Example**: Conduct interviews with nursing staff and patients to gather insights on barriers to effective stroke care and identify themes related to communication, resources, or training.

10. **Performance Metrics Analysis**:
    - **Example**: Analysing metrics such as time-to-treatment for stroke patients to diagnose delays in care processes and areas needing intervention.

These approaches help organisations understand problems deeply and implement targeted solutions for improvement.

22.2 Descriptive analysis

Descriptive analysis involves summarising and interpreting data to provide insights about a particular dataset. Here are some examples across various contexts:

1. **Patient Demographics**:
    - **Example**: A hospital might analyse the age, gender, and ethnicity of stroke patients over the past year to understand the population it serves and tailor prevention programs accordingly.

2. **Clinical Outcomes Summary**:
    - **Example**: Summarizing the average length of stay for stroke patients, the percentage of patients discharged to home versus rehabilitation facilities, and the rates of complications like infections.

3. **Utilisation of Services**:
    - **Example**: Analysing the number of patients treated in the emergency department for strokes by month, highlighting peak times and trends over a year.

4. **Patient Satisfaction Surveys**:
    - **Example**: Calculating average satisfaction scores from patient surveys and categorising feedback on nursing

care, food quality, and discharge processes to identify strengths and areas for improvement.

5. **Financial Metrics**:
   - **Example**: Summarizing the hospital's revenue sources, such as patient care, government funding, and private insurance payments, to provide a comprehensive view of financial health.

6. **Resource Allocation**:
   - **Example**: Analysing the distribution of nursing staff across different units, summarising the ratio of nurses to patients, and identifying units that may be understaffed.

7. **Treatment Protocol Compliance**:
   - **Example**: Summarizing adherence rates to stroke treatment protocols, such as the percentage of eligible patients receiving thrombolysis within the recommended time frame.

8. **Readmission Rates**:
   - **Example**: Analysing the readmission rates for stroke patients within 30 days post-discharge, identifying factors such as age or comorbidities associated with higher rates.

9. **Demographic Trends**:
   - **Example**: Analysing trends in stroke incidence rates by geographic location, gender, or age group over the last decade to identify at-risk populations.

10. **Monthly Performance Reports**:
    - **Example**: Create a report summarising key performance indicators (KPIs) for the stroke unit, including patient turnover rates, average treatment times, and staff performance metrics.

These examples of descriptive analysis help organisations understand current conditions, recognise patterns and inform decision-making processes.

22.3 Predictive analysis

Predictive analysis uses statistical techniques and algorithms to forecast future outcomes based on historical data. Here are some examples across different contexts:

1. **Patient Readmission Prediction**:
   - **Example**: A hospital uses predictive modelling to identify patients at high risk for readmission within 30 days after discharge based on factors such as age, comorbidities, and prior admissions.

2. **Disease Progression Forecasting**:
   - **Example**: Using patient data to predict the progression of chronic diseases like diabetes or heart disease, enabling early interventions to manage health.

3. **Staffing Needs Forecast**:
   - **Example**: Analysing historical patient admission data to predict staffing requirements for nurses and other healthcare professionals, ensuring adequate coverage during peak times.

4. **Patient Outcome Predictions**:
   - **Example**: Developing models to predict outcomes for stroke patients based on initial assessments and treatment protocols, which can help guide treatment decisions.

5. **Appointment No-Show Rates**:
   - **Example**: Analysing past appointment data to predict which patients will most likely miss their scheduled visits, allowing for targeted reminders or follow-ups.

6. **Emergency Room Demand Forecasting**:
   - **Example**: Historical data and seasonal trends are used to predict emergency department patient volumes, helping optimise resource allocation.

7. **Medication Adherence Prediction**:
   - An example is analysing demographic and behavioural data to identify patients at risk of not adhering to prescribed medication regimens, enabling targeted interventions.

8. **Population Health Trends**:
   - **Example**: Predicting and sharing future public health trends and initiatives in a community based on current health data, socioeconomic factors, and environmental conditions.

9. **Frailty Risk Assessment**:
   - **Example**: Using predictive analytics to assess the risk of frailty in elderly patients based on their medical history, mobility data, and social determinants of health.

10. **Cost Forecasting**:
    - An example is analysing historical billing and treatment data to predict future healthcare costs for specific patient populations or treatments, which aids in budget planning.

These examples illustrate how predictive analysis can enhance decision-making in healthcare, improve patient outcomes, and optimise resource management.

22.4 Prescriptive analysis

Prescriptive analysis provides recommendations for actions based on data analysis, often using advanced algorithms and optimisation techniques. Here are some examples across various contexts:

1. **Treatment Recommendations**:
    - **Example**: A healthcare provider uses algorithms to suggest personalised treatment plans for stroke patients based on their medical history, demographics, and clinical guidelines.

2. **Resource Allocation**:
    - **Example**: A hospital employs prescriptive analytics to optimise staff schedules, determining the best nurse-to-patient ratios based on predicted patient volumes and acuity levels.

3. **Supply Chain Management**:
    - **Example**: Data on past usage patterns is used to recommend optimal inventory levels for medical supplies, ensuring that critical items are always in stock while minimising waste.

4. **Risk Management**:
    - **Example**: A predictive model assesses patient risk factors for complications, and prescriptive analysis provides recommendations for pre-emptive interventions or monitoring strategies.

5. **Patient Flow Optimization**:
   - **Example**: Analysing patient admission and discharge patterns to recommend strategies that improve patient throughput and reduce wait times in the emergency department.

6. **Clinical Decision Support**:
   - **Example**: Integrating patient data with clinical guidelines to suggest diagnostic tests or treatments tailored to individual patients enhances physicians' decision-making.

7. **Preventive Care Strategies**:
   - **Example**: Analysing population health data to recommend community health initiatives that target specific groups at high risk for chronic diseases.

8. **Patient Engagement Programs**:
   - **Example**: Using data on patient preferences and behaviours to design targeted communication strategies that encourage adherence to treatment plans.

9. **Financial Forecasting**:
   - An example is a healthcare organisation that uses prescriptive analytics to recommend budget allocations based on predicted service demand and cost trends.

10. **Quality Improvement Initiatives**:
    - **Example**: Analysing clinical performance data to identify areas needing improvement and recommending specific quality improvement projects or training for staff.

These examples demonstrate how prescriptive analysis can guide decision-making in healthcare settings, leading to improved patient outcomes, enhanced operational efficiency, and optimised resource use.

23. Brain Care

Current research shows that the leading causes of brain injuries (clot-based injuries) can be traced to three significant areas:

1. Calcium (furring of veins/arteries),
2. Plaque from teeth and tongue, and
3. Microplastics.
4. Water

23.1 Calcium

Calcium/furring of veins occurs when the diet is poor and underregulated.

(No evidence yet can directly connect brain clots with brain leakages.)

Tip 26

By reducing your intake of fatty foods and eating more vegetables, you can better avoid brain clots and improve brain health.

23.2 Plaque

Plaque builds up on teeth and tongues and then is absorbed and transferred into the bloodstream. These are some of the main contributors to and reasons why clots build up in our veins and brains.

Tip 27

To reduce the amount of plaque in your mouth, clean your teeth at least twice daily (using an electric toothbrush where possible) and remove the plaque from your tongue with a tongue scraper.

23.3 Microplastics

Microplastics within the brain are a recent emerging area of research, and credible research shows that microplastics have been associated directly with Alzheimer's. The study suggests that the brain barrier, the silver that filters foreign parts from the blood, has a problem with cleaning the blood from microplastics. The research suggests that microplastics build up and then shed/tear the veining with the brain, and then patients have black spot/s in their memories.

With this new information and new studies being conducted on brain functionality and the effects of microplastics on the brain, we can only hope that organisations play an active, proactive part in addressing these issues. A few of the steps that could be taken:

- All medications that are prescribed in capsule form with a plastic cover would be changed to avoid plastics.
- All food that uses plastics in their packaging can be changed to new, safer packaging that is safer.
- Plastics used for cups for hot drinks must be changed for safe, not plastic versions.

New studies on microplastics aim to understand micro and macro "absorption" rates, their effects on the body and the brain, and their long-term effects on brain performance. – This is a future area of exploration that requires more research.

It is well understood that cross-contamination within the supply chain can occur when mixed foods and other consumables are transited using plastics. Based on these assumptions, the risk of cross-contamination/harm can be transferred through plastics to humans. – If this has been proven to occur within our food and drink supply chains, why are we allowing medicine producers to produce tablets covered with plastics or microplastics? Where is the government regulation?

(Currently, there are seven main classifications for plastics, and they are not directly monitored or targeted for direct and non-direct harm to humans. Also, the plastics processing organisations are trusted to be self-regulated when significant gaps exist in their research protecting humans.)

23.4 Water

Keep yourself hydrated. Plaque and microplastics have more of a chance of being ejected from the body when you're hydrated. (Not proven scientifically, as yet, or is a method to clean both microplastics and plaque from one's blood; however, dentists, cardio, neuro and phlebotomist (blood) specialists believe that the cause is from contaminated blood and veins.)

Current research is being carried out on in-sleep strokes and how they occur. – The initial finding suggests that there is a connection between in-sleep stroke and patients who have suffered from rehydration. Surprisingly, 20% of all strokes occur in sleep. In 2025 (Jan), 62% of all stroke patients hospitalised suffered from dehydration.

In short, take more water every day. This is a good habit to have.

Tip 28

Have at least 2 pints of water in the morning and another pint of water before sleep.

23.5 Must-have foods

The following is a list of the foods that can help your recovery.

Table 11: Must-have food to improve brain health

Food Names	Reason
Dark chocolate	Help with brain recover
Oily fish	This improves memory, skin, gut health, etc.
Blueberries	Improved mood, memory, gut microbiome and metabolic health.
Eggplant	Good for brain health
Purple and red cabbage	
Red onions	
Purple rice	
Purple sweet potato	
Mulberry	
Red grapes	
Perilla	
Red amaranth	
Plum	
Purple yam	
Eggs	The best source of Choline improves cognitive function.
Beef liver	Improves immune and nervous systems, and strong muscles and gives more energy.
Kiwi fruit	Improves sleep, reduces constipation and improves brain health. Kiwi fruit is good for repairing your brain and DNA.

(Don't more than 1-2 portions each day.)

24. Gifts

To understand the gifts one receives after a stroke or brain injury, one must change one's attitude or perspective on the world. The attitude chapter can help.

I have lost many memories, and some are slowly dripping back to me. Through my research, I have gained more knowledge and upskilled myself in helping others. I view this as a gift. I don't know if I was a bad or a good guy, as I lost my understanding of my previous behaviours/traits that made up my persona. So, with a clean start, I've chosen to be a kind and caring guy who wants to improve the world.

Instead of focusing on what you have lost, I count my blessings.

For example, I think of what I have gained and am grateful for what I regard as my blessing. I have lost people in my journey, e.g. a wife who used me for my money, but I now have a space to have another relationship with someone who loves me. I have lost relationships that have taken me emotionally and financially, and now I have real friends who care and look out for me.

My focus has shifted to my relationships, specifically my children, who are at the top of every list I have. After that, I focused on improving myself and the people who were important to me.

My inner circle of friends has reduced, but the quality of my friends has improved significantly.

I no longer look too far forward and enjoy those present moments that I would have otherwise missed by working. My glass of life is brimming with uncomplicated simplicity and love.

I owe all my actions and mistakes, but I'm more informed and happier this time.

After your brain injury, you will find that you will try some soul searching to understand version 2.0 because it is hard to remember who you were previously, as I lost many of my memories.

The perspective I have chosen to believe in is that the gifts will be advantageous.

The last word on hope is that humans all need connections, purpose, and aims. Hope is a mighty emotion that gives us strength. With self-belief, focus, and determination, you can conquer any obstacle. I have proved this by learning to speak again, writing this book, and helping others talk again. You can succeed, too. However, you must decide what flavour of success you want to chase.

If you doubt what to do, how your actions can be interpreted, or how to look at the brighter side of life, ask yourself what you would do if you had just one day to live. With this attitude, it is easy to be grateful for your blessings, and you will look for the silver linings in every life event.

25. Conclusion

Hospitals are businesses, and their primary aim is to make a profit rather than provide patients with affordable long-term solutions that enable and empower them to help themselves.

This book combines lived experience with the latest scientific research and goes beyond the current practices in any country to offer a long-term strategy for patients. It provides insight into the challenges faced by a brain injury patient with speech difficulties.

The book opens by examining the different types of strokes and their direct effects on a patient's speech.

Next, it examines and dissects the current framework, highlighting its beneficial and detrimental aspects and demonstrating that it is incomplete and inadequate for providing comprehensive speech support throughout the patient's recovery journey.

Having recovered from a stroke, I have recognised significant gaps in the current speech framework and have attempted to address the main end-to-end gaps in an updated framework by consolidating all key global research into this book.

The updated framework I'm proposing is a more straightforward, intuitive end-to-end framework designed to help individuals of all ages improve or regain their speech.

This book stands out because:

- The book adopts a holistic approach to offer extensive recommendations on how to recover beyond traditional treatments.
- The framework included all stakeholders who are directly significant to the patient.
- Enable you, the patient, and support staff to regulate the pace of your assistance.

- It offers a comprehensive end-to-end speech framework that anyone can follow to improve their speech (SCI).
- It enables all stakeholders to transition their planning from short-term strategies to mid- and long-term approaches.
- You are given many tips on how to accelerate recovery. - Tips for expediting your recovery are provided alongside each step in the updated framework.
- Instructs you on how to communicate verbally again following a brain injury.
- It decreases patient recovery time by providing a structured framework that is measurable, trackable, and monitored.
- Reorganise departmental staff resources to prioritise goal setting, performance monitoring, and controlling service delivery costs.
- Reduces the operational costs of providing services to patients, staff, and the organisation.
- Many of the updated framework's items can also be applied in different contexts to help Alzheimer's patients manage their symptoms.

You no longer have to wait for help that may never come, nor do you need to worry about exhausting all your allocated lessons for yourself or your patients. Now, you can offer hope and structured guidance to patients, support staff, and the organisation, positively impacting the delivery and monitoring of speech services during your time in the hospital and beyond.

A key aspect of recovery is the ongoing evaluation of the patient's mindset and attitude. Consider the patient's habits, personal goals, and recovery strategies. In short, you must learn to love yourself again. The person you were before the stroke is quite different from the new version of yourself. Therefore, be kind to yourself and exercise patience with yourself and others.

(This book does not address the issue of depression directly, despite it being a key symptom of any significant and unforeseen major change.

For this book, depression falls outside its scope. However, I have indirectly touched on the subject in the chapters on Tiredness (4), Attitude (5) and Stages of Grief (6).)

The brain functions like a muscle, capable of being retrained when certain parts cease to operate. My colleagues and I have demonstrated that new connections can form to reroute brain signals lost during a stroke. Our brains are truly remarkable, and they can adapt to new challenges. You can relearn and teach anything if you have the necessary time to recover. This is a marathon, not a sprint.

Your biggest nemesis after having a stroke is tiredness. Your brain can be likened to a damaged battery. It struggles to recharge to full power and cannot hold a charge for long. Sleep well and schedule your "thinking and practice" activities for the morning when possible. – Two and a half years after my first stroke, I still need a nap in the afternoon on some days to recharge. This is normal, so be kind to yourself.

Reflecting on the past, I never imagined this would impact me, yet it has. I have become a changed person. Many aspects of my attitude have evolved. I am now more self-aware and attentive to others. I invest time in nurturing and expanding my relationships, and I prioritise better overall health management. To frame these feelings, stroke has allowed me to grow in wonderful ways in directions that I would never have expected to explore or enjoy.

After experiencing a significant health issue, it is entirely natural to feel different. I, too, have faced depression. I had to relearn how to love myself, as much about me has changed. Be patient with everyone, particularly your family, as they remember the person you once were and need time to adjust to this new version of yourself.

I continue to experience both good and bad days. A good day is one when I'm not tired and can clearly express my thoughts, whereas a bad day is when I struggle to find the right words and cannot form a coherent sentence. At present, I'm enjoying more good days than bad, so I have nothing to complain about. Remember, someone else is having a worse day than you, so don't complain about your life; hold on and enjoy the ride.

As I look ahead, I cannot bear to contemplate this happening to me or to anyone I know. Nevertheless, it is bound to occur again. This book will equip you with the tools to customise your speech and comprehension services to suit your individual needs.

Accept that recovering from a brain injury will take time. You must navigate the recovery process in your own way. However, you are not alone. I joined local charity groups to practise speaking and engaging with others who have experienced brain injuries. Additionally, I joined several online stroke groups that have assisted me in managing the various aspects of my recovery and growth. Importantly, I have made many new friends on my recovery journey, as you will also.

As a Hindu, I believe in karma and strive to spread as much love as possible towards the world, as it contributes to making me and this world a better place. If you are in doubt, endeavour to assist someone else, as it replenishes your soul and lifts your spirits.

Get yourself organised as soon as possible. Having a stroke is more about how you react to problems. Are you a fight-or-flight person? I have written my purpose, aims, and routines on my notice board and have a good idea of my habits and those I have yet to adopt. Why the lists? I use lists to help me retrain my learning in a structured, topic-by-topic way.

Possessing this knowledge carries a significant responsibility to assist others. I hope you find it beneficial and share my insights with those around you. Together, we aspire to make this world a better place for everyone. As Mahatma Gandhi stated, *"You must be the change you wish to see in the world."*

Have faith in yourself. Take your recovery at a steady pace. After a few months, I urge you to pause and reflect on how far you have come and how much you have grown. You will be pleasantly surprised. Know I will always be cheering for our shared success.

(If you have enjoyed this book and would like me to create personalised courses, applications, or presentations to assist you, please do not hesitate to contact me directly. I always welcome constructive feedback.

Note: The references can be used as the basis for further development into new treatments and services to help brain injury patients.)

26. List of Tips

Attitude

Tip 1

The above list requires you to stop, understand yourself, and build self-awareness. The secret to mastering yourself is understanding your emotional triggers and how they move your thoughts from a dark to a light place. Practice managing your thoughts by categorising your ideas and then rank your thoughts by category. Also, practice counting backwards from five to zero before speaking.

Also, you can practice giving advice back to another person based on another person's attitude. For example, pick a person you respect and ask yourself what advice they would give to someone else instead if the same question were given to them to answer.

Areas of brain function

Tip 2

Understanding that the senses feed into and out of the brain is crucial. After a stroke or brain injury, the brain has to work overtime to repair itself and help keep the person alive. When I lost my speech, my senses needed time to recalibrate to help me understand the world around me. I found that when my body could not process thoughts or my speech, I would close my eyes to free up other senses/thinking/brain space to allow me to process other activities, e.g. speaking, thinking, etc. – When I closed my eyes and tried to talk, I could speak with little and on issues.

It is essential to understand that when your senses are recalibrating, your body and mind are in a state of flux, and all the senses are uncontrolled. – It feels similar to watching Superman films, and you see when he was a boy and had to use his senses as he adjusted to being on Earth.

Sitting in a quiet room with your thoughts is the best approach to getting used to the new version of yourself.

Tip 3

A few weeks after my stroke, I could not speak sentences at first, but I could bypass the speaking area of my brain and use the singing area to communicate. I would sing simple words.

Tip 4

Find an experienced chiropractor who can unblock and ease your blood flow in and out of your neck and shoulders. This has been crucial in helping me think more clearly and process information.

Tip 5

When one part of the brain is damaged, the brain on the other side that is unaffected has to remap the thoughts from one side to the other. I found that not all of the words were lost. The words had been moved into a long storage space, and it would take me time to remap each map to the new areas in my mind.

Tip 6

When the brain is affected by injury, the brain has difficulty connecting from one side to another. I experimented with weed to test how the effects could help or hinder my thinking. I found that using CBT has little or no positive impact on my speech, whereas when I used THC, my thinking improved, making the connections with me to improve my thinking and my speech. Understand that THC is addictive and should be used in controlled environments only.

Don't give up; start with simple words relevant to your life and build from here.

Easy Framework: "How to Speak Again" / Recording Ability Progress

Tip 7

When recording or updating an ability, please enter the date the patient achieved their level. This enables the patients, support staff, and different organisations to get an overview of the patients in their charge.

Stage 1: Physical Issues / How to Recover?

Tip 8

The following areas will help the patient to recover control of their mouth:

Controlling their swallowing, holding their breath in different parts of the mouth, and their tongue actions. Practice eating using different parts of your mouth to exercise your mouth.

Tip 9

Begin humming.

Tip 10

Sing notes – I picked the most straightforward song I knew and repeated it regularly to exercise my vocal cords.

Tip 11

Create a list of simple words the patient and support team can use to encourage them. The words may not make sense to you, but they will help the patient.

Stage 2: Pictures, Films & Gestures

Tip 12

When you watch TV, switch on the subtitles. This helps your mind connect sounds with letters and your memory. You can enhance your memory recall by remapping your sounds with your mind.

For me and other stroke survivors, our memory has not lost words; instead, it has stored memories in long-term memory. It takes time to remap the brain/mind from one side to the other and re-access memories.

It took me 4-8 times to remember or access the pictures, films, and memories. You have to be very patient at the start, as this is the start of the journey. You will get super tired, as your brain needs time to recover from the new stress (remapping your thoughts, learning sounds and words you had forgotten). I found that at the beginning, I could only be awake for 10-15 minutes before I fell asleep.

Stage 3: Letters, Words, & Numbers

Letter and words

Tip 13

At Levels 2 and 3, I split and broke the words into sounds to make them. Marking or underlining the sounds helped me relearn the words.

Tip 14

Practise putting the words into sentences and into tongue twisters.

Tip 15

Take your time when sounding out the letter in the word. I found that using a phonic dictionary to check words I struggled with.

I found that using the Google Translate program (a free app), you can look up words and get help with their spelling. The apps also allow you to hear the sounds that make up the word and see its phonic spelling.

Tip 16

I practise singing songs, combining my talking and speech abilities. By singing, you bypass the areas of the brain that manage your speech.

(FYI - I only sing behind a closed and locked door because my voice is that flat..)

<u>Numbers</u>

Tip 17

I downloaded a free app called Cross Maths from the Apple App Store to practice and relearn how to apply math functions. The app allows you to select the skill level that applies to you.

<u>Stage 4: Reading & Spoken</u>

Tip 18

The patient can improve their communication ability by slowing down their thinking, varying the speed of delivery, and minimising sensory overloading.

Tip 19

When you start reading again, I suggest reading children's books that use simple words. As you practice, you will improve your spoken words, breath control, and mouth muscles.

Tip 20

While reading the text, I suggest you imagine you are an actor giving a speech.

You can liven up your voice by pretending to be a famous person you can imitate. Please enjoy this stage and remember how far you have come in your recovery. My children love to laugh at me when I make mistakes, reminding me of when I used to read books to them as children before settling them down to bed. Yes, I did the silly voices.

Speaking is one aspect of language, as is listening to the words, so keep this in mind when speaking.

Tip 21

Encourage the patients to imagine themselves in a shop and ask them to describe what they see. Then, repeat this exercise in other environments, such as the gym, garage, airport, recovery groups, or hospital.

How to improve Comprehension

Tip 22

To rebuild the thought categories in your brain again, encourage the patients to imagine they are in a shop and ask them to describe what they see. Then, repeat this exercise in other environments, e.g., the gym, garage, airport, recovery groups, hospital, etc. This is very helpful for stroke and Alzheimer's patients.

I found playing a game called Scattergories very beneficial in helping with memory recall.

Tracking Speech Comprehension / How to use the table

Tip 23

Patient support can periodically re-test the patient to track the development of the support staff and organisations that have been delivered. By updating the abilities and, in turn, the Speech Index, you can identify the areas to focus on with each patient. - This approach can also help the support staff/organisation monitor the delivery performance of services and their effect on their patients.

Overview of Comprehension

Tip 24

Once you take THC, make a list of tasks that you want to focus on, such as practising learning hard-to-say words, sentences, or phases. You will notice a direct improvement in the patient's speech.

Organisations will get a total overview of SCI for each stage. This can help group organisers run cost-efficient focus groups that appeal to patients with similar symptoms. Splitting groups into development stages allows you to deliver/service more patients simultaneously. Patients will readily accept help if they understand and relate to patients with similar speech issues. The journey of regaining one's speech is personal, as is the Speech or Comprehension Index.

The Speech Index can then be compared by patient stage, group, and support staff skill level, and the organisation's recovery rate can provide a simple overview of progress. This simplified approach can help with patient grouping, assigning and allocating resources, and patient processing management.

Effects of CBD and THC

Tip 25

Once you take THC, make a list of tasks that you want to focus on, such as practising learning hard-to-say words, sentences, or phases. You will notice a direct improvement in the patient's speech.

Future of Brain Care

Calcium

Tip 26

By reducing your intake of fatty foods and eating more vegetables, you can better avoid brain clots and improve brain health.

Plaque

Tip 27

To reduce the amount of plaque in your mouth, clean your teeth twice daily (using an electric toothbrush where possible) and remove the plaque from your tongue with a tongue scraper.

Water

Tip 28

Have at least 2 pints of water in the morning and another pint of water before sleep.

27. Tracking Speech & Comprehension - Template

Comprehension Activities	Beginner		Immediate		Fluent
Stage 1: Physical Issues	1	2	3	4	5
Swallowing					
Humming					
Face expressions					
Sounds pitch (Low, medium and high)					
Singing					

Stage 2: Picture, Films & Gestures

Understanding pictures, films and gestures.					
Track the patient's ability to communicate using their dominant hand.					

Stage 3: Letters, Words & Numbers

Track the words you can say (fluently), what you cannot and what is difficult. – This will help you and your support/nurse to focus on the help areas that apply to you.					

Track when the patient can build on the words by applying the words to sentences.				
Track when the patient can use the words to make tongue twisters.				
Track the numbers that you can say and what is more challenging.				
Track the number level that the patient can remember.				
Test the patient with numbers by asking them to recall numbers that increased and decreased in value.				
Test the patient with basic mathematic functions.				

Stage 4: Reading & Spoken

Test 1 (*Gestures*): Measure of accuracy				
Test 1 (*Gestures*): Mental processing speed				
Test 1 (*Gestures*): Speed of delivery				
Test 2 (*Pictures*): Measure of accuracy				
Test 2 (*Pictures*): Mental processing speed				
Test 2 (*Pictures*): Speed of delivery				
Test 3 (*Film*): Measure of accuracy				
Test 3 (*Film*): Mental processing speed				
Test 3 (*Film*): Speed of delivery				

Test 4: Creative speaking with eyes **open**					
Test 4: Creative speaking with eyes **closed**					
Track how the patients can develop their speaking skills:					
Volume – Loud and quiet.					
Register – Nose (high), throat or diaphragm (depth).					
Tibre – Position (Standing or sitting).					
Pace – Talking fast shows excitement, slow is bored or struggling.					
Prosody – The up or down of talking.					
Silence – Appreciate the silence in between topics.					
Test the patient to speak by reading out a book to an audience.					
Test how the patients can group or categorise their thoughts and speech when discussing different topics and environments.					
Test how memory recall works with eyes closed and opened.					

28. References

Aquilani, R., Sessarego, P., Iadarola, P., Barbieri, A. and Boschi, F., 2011. "Nutrition for brain recovery after ischemic stroke: an added value to rehabilitation." *Nutrition in Clinical Practice*, vol.*26, Issue* 3, pp.339-345. DOI.org/10.1177/0884533611405793

Campen M, Nihart A, Garcia M, Liu R, Olewine M, Castillo E, Bleske B, Scott J, Howard T, Gonzalez-Estrella J, Adolphi N, Gallego D, Hayek EE. (2024). "Bioaccumulation of Microplastics in Decedent Human Brains Assessed by Pyrolysis Gas Chromatography-Mass Spectrometry." *Research Square*. DOI: 10.21203/rs.3.rs-4345687/v1.

Cichon, N., Saluk-Bijak, J., Miller, E., Gorniak, L., Redlicka, J., Niwald, M. and Bijak, M., 2021. "The role of supplementation with natural compounds in post-stroke patients.~" *International Journal of molecular sciences*, vol.*22, Issue* 15, p.7893. DOI.org/10.3390/ijms22157893

Giovannini S., Iacovelli C., Loreti C., Lama E., Morciano N., Frisullo G., Biscotti L., Padua L., and Castelli L. (2024). "The role of nutritional supplement on post-stroke fatigue: a pilot randomised controlled trial." The Journal of Nutrition, Health and Aging, vol.28, issue 7, pp. DOI.org.10.1016/j.jnha2024.100256

Kaushik A., Singh A., Gupota, V.K. and Mishra Y.K., (2024). "Nano.microplastic, an invisible threat getting into the brain." Chemosphere, vol.361. DOI.org/10.1016/j.chemosphere.2024.142380

Kay, J., Lesser, R and Coltheart M. (1996). "Psycholinguistic assessments of language processing in aphasia (PALPA): An introduction." *Aphasiology, Vol.10, Issue* 2, pp.159–180. DOI.org/10/10.1080/02687039608248403.

Ncaz (2021) *Dehydration and stroke risk*, *Neurology Consultants of Arizona*. Available at: https://ncaz.org/dehydration-and-stroke-risk/ (Accessed: 31 January 2025).

Rowat, A., Graham, C., and Dennis, M. (2025). "Dehydration in hospital – admitted in patients detection, frequency". *Stroke AHA Journals*, pp.857-9.

Pinto-Grau, M. *et al.* (2020) 'Validation and standardisation of the Psycholinguistic Assessments of Language Processing in Aphasia (PALPA)',

Aphasiology, vol.35 (12), pp. 1593–1610. DOI: 10.1080/02687038.2020.1836317.

Prüst, M., Meijer, J. & Westerink, R.H.S. (2020). "The plastic brain: neurotoxicity of micro- and nanoplastics." *Part Fibre Toxico, vol.*17, Issue 24. DOI.org/10.1186/s12989-020-00358-y

Thompson C.K., Ouden Den D., Bonarkdarpour B., Garibaldi K. and Parrish T. (2010). "Neural plasticity and treatment-induced recovery of sentence processing in agrammatism." *Neuropsychologica*, vol 48, Issue 11, pp. 3211-3227. DOI.org/10.1016/j.neuropsychologia.2010.06.036.

Thumbeck S.M., Schmid P., Chesneau S., Domahs F. (2024). "Efficacy of reading strategies on text-level reading comprehension in people with post-stroke chronic aphasia: A repeated measures study." *Int J Lang Commun Disor*d, vol.59, issue 3, pp.1066-1089. DOI: 10.1111/1460-6984.12983

Van Oers C.A., Vink M., van Zandvoort M.J.E.,van der Worp H.B, De Haan E.H.F., Kappelle, L.J., and Dijhuizen R.M. (2009). "Contribution of the left and right inferior frontal gyrus in recovery from aphasia. A functional MRI study in stroke patients with preserved hemodynamic responsiveness." *Nuerimage* vol.1, Issue 49, pp.885-93. DOI: 10.1016/j.neuroimage.2009.08.057.

Wilson S.M., Eriksson D.K., Brandt T.H., Schneck S.M., Lucanie J.M., Burchfield A.S., Charney S., Quillen I.A., de Riesthal M., Kirshner H.S., Beeson P.M., Ritter L., Kidwell C.S. (2019). "Patterns of Recovery From Aphasia in the First 2 Weeks After Stroke." *J Speech Language Hear Research*, vol.62, Issue 3, pp.723-732. DOI: 10.1044/2018_JSLHR-L-18-0254